SpringerBriefs in Food, Health, and Nutrition

Springer Briefs in Food, Health, and Nutrition present concise summaries of cutting edge research and practical applications across a wide range of topics related to the field of food science, including its impact and relationship to health and nutrition. Subjects include: Food Chemistry, including analytical methods; ingredient functionality; physic-chemical aspects; thermodynamics Food Microbiology, including food safety; fermentation; foodborne pathogens; detection methods Food Process Engineering, including unit operations; mass transfer; heating, chilling and freezing; thermal and non-thermal processing, new technologies Food Physics, including material science; rheology, chewing/mastication Food Policy And applications to: Sensory Science Packaging Food Qualtiy Product Development We are especially interested in how these areas impact or are related to health and nutrition. Featuring compact volumes of 50 to 125 pages, the series covers a range of content from professional to academic. Typical topics might include:

- A timely report of state-of-the art analytical techniques
- A bridge between new research results, as published in journal articles, and a contextual literature review
- A snapshot of a hot or emerging topic
- An in-depth case study
- A presentation of core concepts that students must understand in order to make independent contributions

Bee Ling Tan • Mohd Esa Norhaizan

Nutrients and Oxidative Stress: Biochemistry Aspects and Pharmacological Insights

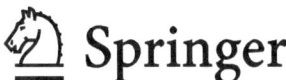 Springer

Bee Ling Tan
Department of Healthcare Professional,
Faculty of Health and Life Sciences
Management and Science University
Shah Alam, Selangor, Malaysia

Mohd Esa Norhaizan
Department of Nutrition, Faculty of
Medicine and Health Sciences
Universiti Putra Malaysia
Serdang, Selangor, Malaysia

ISSN 2197-571X   ISSN 2197-5728   (electronic)
SpringerBriefs in Food, Health, and Nutrition
ISBN 978-3-031-75318-3   ISBN 978-3-031-75319-0   (eBook)
https://doi.org/10.1007/978-3-031-75319-0

This Springer imprint is published by the registered company Springer Nature Switzerland AG
The registered company address is: Gewerbestrasse 11, 6330 Cham, Switzerland

If disposing of this product, please recycle the paper.

Preface

There are different kinds of nutritionally mediated oxidative stress sources that induce inflammation. Emerging research evidence indicates that high consumption of macronutrients can trigger oxidative stress and thereby cause inflammation through nuclear factor-kappa B (NF-κB)-modulated signaling pathways. Dietary fats, animal-based proteins, and carbohydrates are crucial to highlight here because they may contribute to the long-term consequences of nutritionally mediated inflammation. Substantial studies have demonstrated that high-fat and high-glucose diets modulate inflammation, suggesting that oxidative stress may alter the cellular physiological process. Oxidative stress plays a prominent role in the development of numerous human diseases associated with animal-based protein, high-carbohydrate diets, and excessive fat consumption. Obesity represents the main risk factor for chronic diseases, for instance, cardiovascular disease, cancer, and type 2 diabetes. Extensive research highlights the detrimental impacts of diets high in saturated fat and refined carbohydrates. Type 2 diabetes, cardiovascular disease, and obesity are attributed to the sedentary lifestyles, overconsumption of foods high in saturated fats and carbohydrates, and the saturation of nutrient storage. Indeed, the effects of oxidative stress are associated with the absolute quantity and the type of macronutrients; both of these aspects contribute to oxidative stress and may favor the development of obesity-associated diseases and obesity. Nonetheless, the underlying mechanisms of nutritionally mediated oxidative stress are complex and poorly understood. Based on our knowledge, the literature reported on nutritionally mediated oxidative stress and the role of diets in oxidative stress-induced diseases has not well been compiled in the form of a brief/book. Indeed, this disintegrated literature needs to be compiled together to deliver information at one point. Hence, this book attempts to explore how dietary choices dampen or exacerbate inflammation and oxidative stress. The implications of oxidative stress in glucose metabolism and adipocyte and obesity-associated non-communicable diseases are also discussed in this book. This book covers several issues linked to nutritionally mediated oxidative stress, including high carbohydrates, high animal-based proteins, and excessive consumption of fats and oxidative stress, and molecular mechanisms of oxidative stress-induced diseases. The role of diets in oxidative stress-induced diseases is also discussed in this book. By summarizing all the literature cohesively and lucidly in one book/brief, it would provide a cohesive representation of the information and practical reference on the underlying mechanisms of nutritionally mediated oxidative stress involved in the prevention of chronic diseases for the allied stakeholders and readers. A better understanding of the nutritionally mediated oxidative stress and the molecular mechanisms of oxidative stress in the development of chronic diseases and obesity would provide a useful approach. This is because oxidative stress can be modulated by both intrinsic and extrinsic factors, thereby providing a plausible means to prevent metabolic ailments.

Shah Alam, Selangor, Malaysia   Bee Ling Tan

Contents

Chapter 1
Introduction and Background

Nutrition and diet influence both the harmful and beneficial aspects of oxidative processes (Sharma and Mehdi 2023). Various sources of nutritionally mediated oxidative stress induce inflammation. Oxidative stress plays a crucial role in the development of a wide range of human diseases (Tan et al. 2018a). Reactive nitrogen species (RNS) and reactive oxygen species (ROS) are continuously generated in the body through mitochondrial bioenergetics, oxidative metabolism, and immune function (Tan et al. 2018b). The detrimental effects of free radicals from ROS and RNS result in potential biological damage, leading to oxidative stress and nitrosative stress, respectively (Engwa et al. 2022). The mitochondrion is the crucial cell organelle in ROS generation (Popov 2023). It produces adenosine triphosphate (ATP) through a series of oxidative phosphorylation processes. The most frequent forms of ROS including hydroxyl radical, singlet oxygen, hyphochlorous acid, lipid peroxides, hypochlorite, hydrogen peroxide, and superoxide anion, which are involved in the growth, death, differentiation, and progression of cells (Tan and Norhaizan 2021). They can bind with proteins, enzymes, membrane lipids, nucleic acids, and other small molecules. Indeed, short-term postprandial mitochondrial oxidative stress contributes to inflammation, which is predominantly modulated by nuclear factor-kappa B (NF-κB). By contrast, long-term chronic overconsumption leads to obesity, which triggers permanent states of inflammation through the production of white adipose tissue which secretes proinflammatory factors (Tan et al. 2018b). Compelling evidence has demonstrated that a high-fat and high-glucose diet causes inflammation, suggesting that oxidative stress may affect cellular physiological processes (Tan et al. 2018b; Tan and Norhaizan 2019).

Extensive research reveals the detrimental impacts of diets high in refined carbohydrates and saturated fat (Taylor et al. 2021). Cardiovascular disease (CVD), type 2 diabetes, and obesity are attributed to the saturation of nutrient storage, overconsumption of foods high in saturated fats and carbohydrates, and sedentary lifestyles (Hariharan et al. 2022). A study reported by Park et al. (2016) examined the impact of a Westernized dietary pattern on inflammatory diseases, such as colorectal cancer, and consistently demonstrated a similar trend. The study highlighted the fundamental concept that diet quality can influence systemic inflammation and immune function.

The prevalence of obesity has nearly tripled between 1975 and 2016 worldwide (Boutari and Mantzoros 2022), mainly due to the sedentary lifestyle and intake of unhealthy diets such as refined carbohydrates and high sugar diets. In addition, environmental, metabolic, endocrine, and genetic factors are also considered the primary common causes of obesity in the last decades (Upadhyay et al. 2018; Polyzos and Mantzoros 2019). Specifically, the prevalence of global obesity has risen about 2% points per decade (NCD Risk Factor Collaboration 2017). According to the World Health Organization (2023), more than 1 billion people worldwide are obese, including 39 million children, 340 million adolescents, and 650 million adults. By 2025, nearly 167 million adults and children are expected to become less healthy due to being overweight or obese (World Health Organization 2023). Individuals who are overweight or obese have an increased risk of developing cancer, stroke, hypertension, CVD, type 2 diabetes, coronary heart disease, and inflammatory disorders.

The effects of oxidative stress are associated with their absolute quantity and the type of macronutrients consumed (Tan and Norhaizan 2021), both of these aspects may favor the development of obesity-related non-communicable diseases and obesity as well as contribute to oxidative stress (Nouripour et al. 2021). Nonetheless, the underlying mechanisms of action of nutritionally mediated oxidative stress are complex and are worth discussing further.

To the best of the authors' knowledge, the literature on nutritionally mediated oxidative stress and the role of diets in oxidative stress-induced diseases has not been thoroughly compiled into a single brief or book. Fragmented knowledge needs to be consolidated to provide comprehensive information in one source. Therefore, this book attempts to discuss several issues related to nutrients and oxidative stress, including elements of fundamentals of oxidative metabolism, nutritionally mediated oxidative stress, molecular mechanisms of oxidative stress-induced diseases, high carbohydrates intake and type 2 diabetes, high animal-based proteins and cancer, excessive consumption of fats and cardiovascular disease, the role of food sources in oxidative stress-induced diseases, and future prospects.

References

Boutari C, Mantzoros CS (2022) A 2022 update on the epidemiology of obesity and a call to action: as its twin COVID-19 pandemic appears to be receding, the obesity and dysmetabolism pandemic continues to rage on. Metabolism 133:155217

Engwa GA, Nweke FN, Nkeh-Chungag BN (2022) Free radicals, oxidative stress-related diseases and antioxidant supplementation. Altern Ther Health Med 28:114–128

Hariharan R, Odjidja EN, Scott D et al (2022) The dietary inflammatory index, obesity, type 2 diabetes, and cardiovascular risk factors and diseases. Obes Rev 23:e13349

NCD Risk Factor Collaboration (NCD-RisC) (2017) Worldwide trends in body-mass index, underweight, overweight, and obesity from 1975 to 2016: a pooled analysis of 2416 population-based measurement studies in 128·9 million children, adolescents, and adults. Lancet (London, England) 390:2627–2642

Nouripour F, Mazloom Z, Fararouei M et al (2021) Effect of protein and carbohydrate distribution among meals on quality of life, sleep quality, inflammation, and oxidative stress in patients with type 2 diabetes: a single-blinded randomized controlled trial. Food Sci Nutr 9:6176–6185

Park Y, Lee J, Oh JH et al (2016) Dietary patterns and colorectal cancer risk in a Korean population: a case-control study. Medicine 95:article e3759

Polyzos SA, Mantzoros CS (2019) Obesity: seize the day, fight the fat. Metabolism 92:1–5

Popov L-D (2023) Mitochondria as intracellular signalling organelles. An update. Cell Signal 109:110794

Sharma V, Mehdi MM (2023) Oxidative stress, inflammation and hormesis: the role of dietary and lifestyle modifications on aging. Neurochem Int 164:105490

Tan BL, Norhaizan ME (2019) Effect of high-fat diets on oxidative stress, cellular inflammatory response and cognitive function. Nutrients 11:2579

Tan BL, Norhaizan ME (2021) Oxidative stress, diet and prostate cancer. World J Mens Health 39:195–207

Tan BL, Norhaizan ME, Liew W-P-P et al (2018a) Antioxidant and oxidative stress: a mutual interplay in age-related diseases. Front Pharmacol 9:1162

Tan BL, Norhaizan ME, Liew W-P-P (2018b) Nutrients and oxidative stress: friend or foe? Oxid Med Cell Longev 2018., Article ID 9719584:24

Taylor ZB, Stevenson RJ, Ehrenfeld L et al (2021) The impact of saturated fat, added sugar and their combination on human hippocampal integrity and function: a systematic review and meta-analysis. Neurosci Biobehav Rev 130:91–106

Upadhyay J, Farr O, Perakakis N et al (2018) Obesity as a disease. Med Clin North Am 102:13–33

World Health Organization (2023) World Obesity Day 2022 – Accelerating action to stop obesity. https://www.who.int/news/item/04-03-2022-world-obesity-day-2022-accelerating-action-to-stop-obesity. Accessed on 9 Feb 2023

Chapter 2
Elements of Fundamentals of Oxidative Metabolism

Redox homeostasis and oxidative metabolism have been demonstrated as an integral part of aerobic life (Commoner et al. 1954). Under unfavorable cellular circumstances, oxygen derivatives can interrupt oxidative equilibrium and thereby result in the damage of proteins, lipids, and nucleic acids, and compromise cell viability (Halliwell 1991).

Compelling evidence has revealed that oxidative stress lies in the pathophysiological core of a plethora of human diseases (Kaur et al. 2021; Salekeen et al. 2022). Nonetheless, under physiological conditions or normal functions of the human body, for instance, nutrition can potentially produce oxidative stress. Macronutrients can be inflammatory and may serve as a pro-oxidant (Tan et al. 2018).

2.1 Oxidative Stress: A Brief Description

There are two primary categories of oxidants or free radicals: reactive nitrogen species (RNS) and reactive oxygen species (ROS) (Jomova et al. 2023). ROS derived from molecular oxygen is produced upon incomplete reaction of oxygen such as hydrogen peroxide (H_2O_2), hydroxyl radical (OH^-), singlet oxygen, and superoxide anion (O_2^-) (Singh 2022). This activation takes place in several cellular processes (Fig. 2.1). The harmful effects of free RNS and ROS can lead a potential biological damage, namely nitrosative stress and oxidative stress, respectively (Singh et al. 2022). Oxidative stress is regarded as an imbalance between anti- and prooxidant species, which causes cellular and molecular damage (Pisoschi et al. 2021). Mitochondria are the predominant cell organelle in ROS generation via oxidative phosphorylation processes to produce adenosine triphosphate (ATP), a molecule that is important for cellular actions (Weinberg et al. 2015). The electron transport chain consumes about 90% of the total oxygen (O_2) taken up by the cells (Wallace

© The Author(s), under exclusive license to Springer Nature Switzerland AG 2024
B. L. Tan, M. E. Norhaizan, *Nutrients and Oxidative Stress: Biochemistry Aspects and Pharmacological Insights*, SpringerBriefs in Food, Health, and Nutrition, https://doi.org/10.1007/978-3-031-75319-0_2

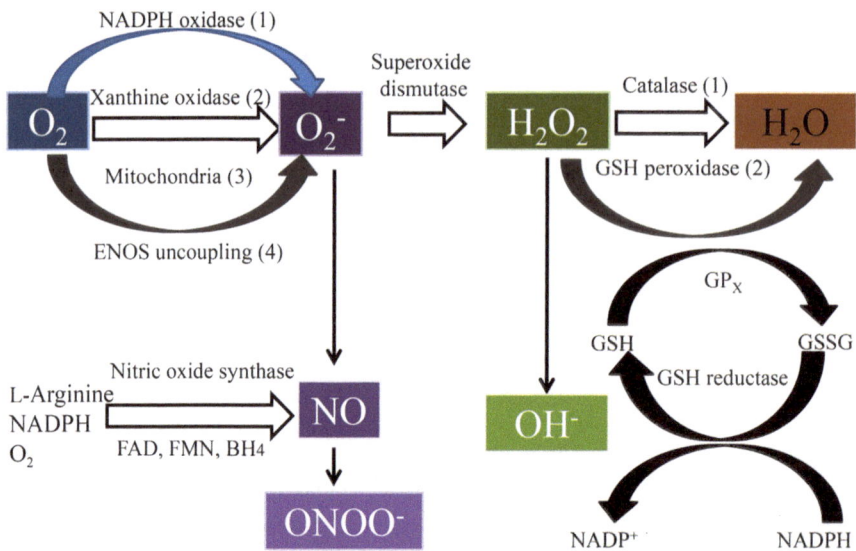

Fig. 2.1 Molecular pathways of reactive nitrogen species (RNS) and reactive oxygen species (ROS) production and clearance via different enzymatic reactions. *BH4* tetrahydrobiopterin, *ENOS* endothelial nitric oxide synthase, *FAD* flavin adenine dinucleotide, *FMN* flavin mononucleotide, *GPx* glutathione peroxidases, *GSH* glutathione, *GSSG* glutathione disulfide, H_2O_2 hydrogen peroxide, *NADPH* nicotinamide adenine dinucleotide phosphate, *NO* nitric oxide, *RNS* reactive nitrogen species, *ROS* reactive oxygen species, O_2^- superoxide anion, OH^- hydroxyl radical, $ONOO^-$ peroxynitrite. (Source: Droge 2002)

2013). During this process, ROS are produced as a by-product for the partial four-electron reduction of O_2 to generate water molecules, which is the last electron acceptor in the ATP production process (Ambrosio et al. 1993). In the normal physiological states, approximately 0.1–0.5% of inhaled O_2 is converted to superoxide (O_2^-) (Servais et al. 2009). The oxidation and production of ROS occur in a controlled manner during the normal healthy state. On the other hand, the ROS generation is elevated under a disease state or high-stress condition. The ROS produced from aerobic respiration contributed a cumulative oxidative damage in macromolecules such as DNA, lipids, and proteins, thereby leading to cell death (Checa and Aran 2020), and influencing the healthspan of many crucial organ systems (Akbari et al. 2019).

Oxygen free radicals such as hydroxyl radical ($OH^{•-}$), superoxide anion radical ($O_2^{•-}$), and alkyl peroxyl radical ($^{•}OOCR$), are potent initiators in lipid peroxidation, the role of which is well-established in the pathogenesis of diseases (Bhatti et al. 2022). Upon lipid peroxidation is activated, a propagation of chain reactions will take place until termination products are generated (Farhoosh 2022). Hence, end products of lipid peroxidation such as 4-hydroxy-2-nonenol (4-HNE), F2-isoprostanes, and malondialdehyde (MDA), are accumulated in biological systems (Mas-Bargues et al. 2021; Trares et al. 2022; Zhang et al. 2022). DNA bases are prone to ROS oxidation, and the primary detectable oxidation product of DNA bases is 8-hydroxy-2-deoxyguanosine (Shekaftik and Nasirzadeh 2021). The oxidation of DNA bases can lead to deletions and mutations in both mitochondrial and nuclear DNA. In general, mitochondrial DNA is relatively susceptible to oxidative damage due to its deficient repair capacity and proximity to ROS compared to nuclear DNA (Muftuoglu et al. 2014). These oxidative alterations result in functional changes in enzymatic and structural proteins, which subsequently contribute to substantial physiological impact (Xiong and Guo 2021). Furthermore, redox modulations of transcription factors also decrease or increase their specific DNA binding activities hence mediating gene expression (Dimauro et al. 2020).

2.2 Nitrosative Stress

RNS is a family of chemical compounds that are derived from nitric oxide (NO) (Al-Shehri 2021). Under physiological conditions, NO is synthesized from L-arginine through the catalytic action of nitric oxide synthase (NOS) with the presence of catalytic cofactors, flavin mononucleotide (FMN), flavin adenine dinucleotide, and tetrahydrobiopterin (BH4). Under certain stimuli, NO reacts with superoxide to produce peroxynitrite ($ONOO^-$), which is believed to be one of the most toxic RNS generated in the body and subsequently stimulates the generation of other forms of RNS including dinitrogen trioxide (N_2O_3) and nitrogen dioxide ($\bullet NO_2$) (Pacher et al. 2007). The major form of RNS includes peroxynitrite ($ONOO-$) and nitric oxide (NO) (Kwon et al. 2021). When excess NO is present, this process causes the formation of nitrogen dioxide radicals. Higher concentration of NO leads to the formation of N_2O_3, and subsequently results in nitrosation (Ford and Miranda 2020).

In addition to the prooxidants mentioned above, other molecules such as advanced glycation end products (AGEs) have also shown prooxidant and inflammatory properties (Salazar et al. 2021). AGEs or glycotoxins, comprised a heterogenous group of more than 20 different compounds, derived from endogenous nonenzymatic glycation of macromolecules or from absorbed exogenous sources. Upon formation, AGEs stimulate the formation of RNS and ROS via several signaling pathways (Cepas et al. 2020). The binding of AGEs to their multi-ligand receptor for advanced glycation end products (RAGE) stimulates NF-κB, subsequently leading to increased ROS production and NADPH oxidase activation (Muthyalaiah et al. 2021).

Antioxidants control autoxidation by inhibiting the formation of free radicals or by interfering with the propagation of free radicals via a few mechanisms. These compounds facilitate the quenching $\bullet$ O_2^-, scavenging the species that initiate the peroxidation, preventing the formation of peroxides, and breaking the autoxidative chain reaction (Umber et al. 2023). The most effective antioxidants are those exerting an ability to interrupt the free radical chain reaction. They possess aromatic or phenolic rings which allow these antioxidants to donate H$\bullet$ to the free radicals produced during oxidation. The radical intermediate is subsequently stabilized by the resonance delocalization of the electron within the aromatic ring (Romero et al. 2018). When high production of free radicals cannot be compensated by the antioxidant defense system of the body, ROS initiated via several molecular pathways and oxidative stress dominates (Chung et al. 2021).

2.3 Free Radical and Nonradical Oxidants

Both 2-electron (nonradical) and 1-electron (free radical) transfer reactions occur in biological systems, in which disruption of either can cause oxidative stress (Girotti and Korytowski 2023). Indeed, free radicals are unstable and reactive molecules leading to a chain reaction of oxidation. Despite free radical reactions have been a common target in oxidative stress studies, research evidence revealed that scavenging mechanisms in biological systems limit propagation under certain circumstances, whereas the non-radical reactions predominate under most oxidative stress conditions (Munteanu and Apetrei 2021). Nonradical oxidants such as disulfides, reactive sulfur species, and H_2O_2, and several common metabolites have quinone and carbonyl structures (Martemucci et al. 2022). Furthermore, O_2 and other chemicals can exist in activated states with electron pairs or electrons in orbitals other than the ground state (Dennis et al. 2019). For O_2, this is termed singlet oxygen ($^1O_2$) which can be formed as a consequence of chemical reactions or due to stimulation by visible light in the presence of photosensitizers. Indeed, the activated chemicals, for instance, $^1O_2$ are far more reactive with biomolecules compared to ground-state O_2 and contribute to oxidative stress (Dennis et al. 2019).

2.4 Redox Theory and Oxidative Stress Mechanisms

Advances in redox theory give a framework to highlight the mode of actions of oxidative stress inclusive of the range of dietary oxidants and interacting antioxidant systems (Jones and Sies 2015). Several primary advances result from studies of the NADPH oxidase (NOX) family of enzymes. These are commonly distributed among different types of cells (Lambeth 2004; Griendling 2006) and cause the production of superoxide anion radical ($O_2^{-\bullet}$) and maintenance of steady-state H_2O_2 concentration in the low nanomolar range (Sies 2017). Evaluation of these systems demonstrated that in combination with thioredoxin (TRX)- and GSH peroxidase-dependent peroxiredoxins, NADPH-dependent systems function in opposition to concomitantly with H_2O_2 production and elimination. Therefore, this creates a fail-safe system to maintain an oxidant tone in cells. Reduction in NADPH limits the reactions for both oxidant elimination and oxidant production. Subsequently, the parallel of NAD and NADP systems allows catabolism and anabolism to occur simultaneously in cells (Sies 1982). The maintenance of steady-state pools of oxidants and reductants allows oxidative and reductive metabolism to occur simultaneously in cells. This is further elaborated in a redox control structure which modulates the redox state of protein cysteine (Cys) residues in functionally associated proteins (Jones and Go 2011; Go et al. 2015). Indeed, the redox organizational structure allows a wide range of functional systems to be coordinated via redox control of thiol sulfur to switch in proteins (Schafer and Buettner 2001) and maintains a relatively stable of these systems against both reductants and oxidants. Redox signaling occurs within this structure by stimulation of NOX enzymes in certain specific subcellular sites by creating localized oxidant gradients (Brown and Griendling 2009).

2.5   Redox States of Intracellular Compartments

Mitochondria are the main hubs of energy generation, using oxygen as the final electron acceptor, and utilizing the electron transport chain as a means of generating ATP. Glutathione (GSH) system and mitochondrial thioredoxin are maintained at a relatively reducing steady-state level, which demonstrates a need for powerful defenses against a range of oxidative and reductive forces among redox couples. Mitochondria possess unique redox-related transporters and enzymes serving in this protection, for instance, glutaredoxin 2, which plays a vital role in protecting from apoptosis and oxidative stress and catalyzing reversible oxidation and glutathionylation of mitochondrial membrane proteins (Garcia et al. 2010).

The nuclear redox state is relatively low with translocation of Trx1 into nuclei toward oxidative stress. Many transcriptional factors such as NF-κB, p53, and Nrf2 exert redox-sensitive cysteine residues in the DNA-binding region, providing nuclear redox control as well as cytoplasmic stimulation of signaling cascades toward oxidative stress (Nagini et al. 2021). A study evaluated the thiol-dependent antioxidant systems in subcellular regions of human colonic epithelial HT-29 cells following the depletion of glutamine, glucose, and energy precursors in the culture medium demonstrated that mitochondrial Trx2 and cytosolic Trx1 were oxidized without nuclear Trx1 oxidation (Go et al. 2007).

The endoplasmic reticulum exerts unique enzyme systems to support the introduction of disulfide bonds for the proper folding of proteins in secretion (Victor et al. 2021). This system maintains an oxidized state relative to the cytoplasm, and disruption by either oxidizing or reducing environment may result in cell death, endoplasmic reticulum stress, and aberrant protein folding in the secretory pathways. Peroxisomes and H_2O_2 —producing enzymes with lysosomes and degradation organelle and endocytosis turnover products are also relatively oxidizing (Walker et al. 2018). Substantial studies highlight that organelles exert a broad spectrum of functions and are comprised of several redox systems operating in a dynamic steady level to support specific functions (Sies et al. 2022; Lee and Loscalzo 2020).

2.6 Plasma and Extracellular Redox State

A holistic network model for oxidative stress emphasizes the differences of redox systems in the body systems and addresses the mixed effects of dietary interventions on global oxidative stress (Feelisch et al. 2022). Organ systems communicate via the plasma and thus the plasma redox measures give both a practical approach and a conceptual connectivity to link human health, oxidative stress, and diet. Research evidence has suggested that dietary factors, for instance, glutamine and sulfur amino acid (SAA) intakes are related to plasma redox state (Pajares and Pérez-Sala 2018). The study further showed an association between human mid-brain glutamate and dietary SAA using magnetic resonance spectroscopy (Park et al. 2012).

2.7 Intraorgan Redox Control

Some studies have emerged to highlight the extent of redox variations in several regions of organs. Higher concentrations of GSH are found in crypts in intestinal epithelia and rapidly growing regions of tumors (Dennis et al. 2019). Glutathione (GSH) contents also differ among different cell types such as bone marrow niche, lungs, brain, and other organs, and thereby local differences are expected based on the types of cells. The pancreas is a specific organ for examining the redox variations due to the regionally distinct exocrine and endocrine functions. Redox signaling is a vital component that modulates the normal insulin release from β-cells. Oxidative stress is associated with the dysfunction of β-cells and the risk of type 2 diabetes (Dludla et al. 2023). The high diversity of cell types and endocrine activities within the pancreatic islets of Langerhans allows evaluation of how the interplay of redox signaling affects disrupted and normal functioning.

Thiol/disulfide redox control in the extracellular space was previously reported by Moriarty-Craige and Jones (2004). It has been demonstrated its function in maintaining the redox status of thiols in transporters, receptors, and integrins in the cell membrane. A study reported by Sies and Graf (1985) demonstrated that α-adrenergic agonists activated GSH release. Consistent with the study reported by Sies and Graf (1985), α-adrenergic agonists have also been reported to stimulate GSH transport in the small intestine (Hagen et al. 1991; Bai and Jones 1996). Evidence from these studies suggests that circulating factors associated with plasma redox systems and stress hormones may affect the homeostatic mechanisms for plasma GSH.

The modulation of extracellular E_hCySS in *in vitro* was enhanced by growth factors such as insulin-like growth factor-1 (IGF-1) and epidermal growth factor (EGF) (Jonas et al. 2002). The rates of thiol efflux were activated by high perfusate glutathione disulfide (GSSG) in perfused rat intestines (Dahm and Jones 1994). These data suggest that a humoral redox control system may operate to maintain systemic plasma E_hCySS and E_hGSSG. In this regard, the regulation of the interorgan control system may account for the changes in redox potential accompanying aging, obesity, and inflammation. This system would effectively parallel with humoral systems controlling blood CO_2, blood O_2, blood pH, and blood glucose. Collectively, this system may be essential given that $E_h GSSG$ controls platelet activation and $E_h CySS$ modulates inflammatory signaling.

References

Akbari M, Kirkwood TBL, Bohr VA (2019) Mitochondria in the signaling pathways that control longevity and health span. Ageing Res Rev 54:100940

Al-Shehri SS (2021) Reactive oxygen and nitrogen species and innate immune response. Biochimie 181:52–64

Ambrosio G, Zweier JL, Duilio C et al (1993) Evidence that mitochondrial respiration is a source of potentially toxic oxygen free radicals in intact rabbit hearts subjected to ischemia and reflow. J Biol Chem 268:18532–18541

Bai C, Jones DP (1996) GSH transport and GSH-dependent detoxication in small intestine of rats exposed *in vivo* to hypoxia. Am J Phys 271:G701–G706

Bhatti JS, Sehrawat A, Mishra J et al (2022) Oxidative stress in the pathophysiology of type 2 diabetes and related complications: current therapeutics strategies and future perspectives. Free Radical Biol Med 184:114–134

Brown DI, Griendling KK (2009) NOX proteins in signal transduction. Free Radical Biol Med 47:1239–1253

Cepas V, Collino M, Mayo JC et al (2020) Redox signaling and advanced glycation end products (AGEs) in diet-related diseases. Antioxidants 9:142

Checa J, Aran JM (2020) Reactive oxygen species: drivers of physiological and pathological processes. J Inflamm Res 13:1057–1073

Chung J, Huda MN, Shin Y et al (2021) Correlation between oxidative stress and transforming growth factor-beta in cancers. Int J Mol Sci 22:13181

Commoner B, Townsend J, Pake GE (1954) Free radicals in biological materials. Nature 174:689–691

Dahm LJ, Jones DP (1994) Clearance of glutathione disulfide from rat mesenteric vasculature. Toxicol Appl Pharmacol 129:272–282

Dennis KK, Go Y-M, Jones DP (2019) Redox systems biology of nutrition and oxidative stress. J Nutr 149:553–565

Dimauro I, Paronetto MP, Caporossi D (2020) Exercise, redox homeostasis and the epigenetic landscape. Redox Biol 35:101477

Dludla PV, Mabhida SE, Ziqubu K et al (2023) Pancreatic β-cell dysfunction in type 2 diabetes: implications of inflammation and oxidative stress. World J Diabetes 14:130–146

Droge W (2002) Free radicals in the physiological control of cell function. Physiol Rev 82:47–95

Farhoosh R (2022) New insights into the kinetic and thermodynamic evaluations of lipid peroxidation. Food Chem 375:131659

Feelisch M, Cortese-Krott MM, Santolini J et al (2022) Systems redox biology in health and disease. EXCLI J 21:623–646

Ford PC, Miranda KM (2020) The solution chemistry of nitric oxide and other reactive nitrogen species. Nitric Oxide 103:31–46

Garcia J, Han D, Sancheti H et al (2010) Regulation of mitochondrial glutathione redox status and protein glutathionylation by respiratory substrates. J Biol Chem 285:39646–39654

Girotti AW, Korytowski W (2023) Trafficking of oxidative stress-generated lipid hydroperoxides: pathophysiological implications. Free Radic Res 57:130–139

Go YM, Ziegler TR, Johnson JM et al (2007) Selective protection of nuclear thioredoxin-1 and glutathione redox systems against oxidation during glucose and glutamine deficiency in human colonic epithelial cells. Free Radic Biol Med 42:363–370

Go YM, Chandler JD, Jones DP (2015) The cysteine proteome. Free Radic Biol Med 84:227–245

Griendling KK (2006) NADPH oxidases: new regulators of old functions. Antioxid Redox Signal 8:1443–1445

Hagen TM, Bai C, Jones DP (1991) Stimulation of glutathione absorption in rat small intestine by alpha-adrenergic agonists. FASEB J 5:2721–2727

Halliwell B (1991) Reactive oxygen species in living systems: source, biochemistry, and role in human disease. Am J Med 91:14S–22S

Jomova K, Raptova R, Alomar SY et al (2023) Reactive oxygen species, toxicity, oxidative stress, and antioxidants: chronic diseases and aging. Arch Toxicol 97:2499–2574

Jonas CR, Ziegler TR, Gu LH et al (2002) Extracellular thiol/disulfide redox state affects proliferation rate in a human colon carcinoma (Caco2) cell line. Free Radic Biol Med 33:1499–1506

Jones DP, Go YM (2011) Mapping the cysteine proteome: analysis of redox-sensing thiols. Curr Opin Chem Biol 15:103–112

Jones DP, Sies H (2015) The redox code. Antioxid Redox Signal 23:734–746

Kaur G, Sharma A, Bhatnagar A (2021) Role of oxidative stress in pathophysiology of rheumatoid arthritis: insights into NRF2-KEAP1 signalling. Autoimmunity 54:385–397

Kwon N, Kim D, Swamy KMK et al (2021) Metal-coordinated fluorescent and luminescent probes for reactive oxygen species (ROS) and reactive nitrogen species (RNS). Coord Chem Rev 427:213581

Lambeth JD (2004) NOX enzymes and the biology of reactive oxygen. Nat Rev Immunol 4:181–189

Lee LY, Loscalzo J (2020) Chapter 3 – Systems biology and network medicine: an integrated approach to redox biology and pathobiology. In: Sies H (ed) Oxidative stress: eustress and distress, pp 29–49

Martemucci G, Costagliola C, Mariano M et al (2022) Free radical properties, source and targets, antioxidant consumption and health. Oxygen 2:48–78

Mas-Bargues C, Escrivá C, Dromant M et al (2021) Lipid peroxidation as measured by chromatographic determination of malondialdehyde. Human plasma reference values in health and disease. Arch Biochem Biophys 709:108941

Moriarty-Craige SE, Jones DP (2004) Extracellular thiols and thiol/disulfide redox in metabolism. Annu Rev Nutr 24:481–509

Muftuoglu M, Mori MP, de Souza-Pinto NC (2014) Formation and repair of oxidative damage in the mitochondrial DNA. Mitochondrion 17:164–181

Munteanu IG, Apetrei C (2021) Analytical methods used in determining antioxidant activity: a review. Int J Mol Sci 22:3380

Muthyalaiah YS, Jonnalagadda B, John CM et al (2021) Impact of Advanced Glycation End products (AGEs) and its receptor (RAGE) on cancer metabolic signaling pathways and its progression. Glycoconj J 38:717–734

Nagini S, Thiyagarajan P, Rao KS (2021) Interplay between reactive oxygen species and key players in the DNA damage response signaling network. In: Chakraborti S, Ray BK, Roychowdhury S (eds) Handbook of oxidative stress in cancer: mechanistic aspects. Springer, Singapore, pp 1–18

Pacher P, Beckman JS, Liaudet L (2007) Nitric oxide and peroxynitrite in health and disease. Physiol Rev 87:315–424

Pajares MA, Pérez-Sala D (2018) Mammalian Sulphur amino acid metabolism: a nexus between redox regulation, nutrition, epigenetics, and detoxification. Antioxid Redox Signal 29:408–452

Park Y, Zhao T, Miller NG et al (2012) Sulfur amino acid-free diet results in increased glutamate in human midbrain: a pilot magnetic resonance spectroscopic study. Nutrition 28:235–241

Pisoschi AM, Pop A, Iordache F et al (2021) Oxidative stress mitigation by antioxidants – an overview on their chemistry and influences on health status. Eur J Med Chem 209:112891

Romero KJ, Galliher MS, Pratt DA et al (2018) Radicals in natural product synthesis. Chem Soc Rev 47:7851–7866

Salazar J, Navarro C, Ortega Á et al (2021) Advanced glycation end products: new clinical and molecular perspectives. Int J Environ Res Public Health 18:7236

Salekeen R, Haider AN, Akhter F et al (2022) Lipid oxidation in pathophysiology of atherosclerosis: current understanding and therapeutic strategies. Int J Cardiol Cardiovasc Risk Prev 14:200143

Schafer FQ, Buettner GR (2001) Redox environment of the cell as viewed through the redox state of the glutathione disulfide/glutathione couple. Free Radic Biol Med 30:1191–1212

Servais S, Boussouar A, Molnar A et al (2009) Age-related sensitivity to lung oxidative stress during ozone exposure. Free Radic Res 39:305–316

Shekaftik SO, Nasirzadeh N (2021) 8-Hydroxy-2′-deoxyguanosine (8-OHdG) as a biomarker of oxidative DNA damage induced by occupational exposure to nanomaterials: a systematic review. Nanotoxicology 15:850–864

Sies H (1982) Nicotinamide nucleotide compartmentation. In: Sies H (ed) Metabolic compartmentation. Academic, New York, pp 205–231

Sies H (2017) Hydrogen peroxide as a central redox signaling molecule in physiological oxidative stress: oxidative eustress. Redox Biol 11:613–619

Sies H, Graf P (1985) Hepatic thiol and glutathione efflux under the influence of vasopressin, phenylephrine and adrenaline. Biochem J 226:545–549

Sies H, Belousov VV, Chandel NS et al (2022) Defining roles of specific reactive oxygen species (ROS) in cell biology and physiology. Nat Rev Mol Cell Biol 23:499–515

Singh D (2022) Juggling with reactive oxygen species and antioxidant defense system–a coping mechanism under salt stress. Plant Stress 5:100093

Singh A, Kukreti R, Saso L et al (2022) Mechanistic insight into oxidative stress-triggered signaling pathways and type 2 diabetes. Molecules 27:950

Tan BL, Norhaizan ME, Liew W-P-P (2018) Nutrients and oxidative stress: friend or foe? Oxid Med Cell Longev 2018., Article ID 9719584:24

Trares K, Chen L-J, Schöttker B (2022) Association of F2-isoprostane levels with Alzheimer's disease in observational studies: a systematic review and meta-analysis. Ageing Res Rev 74:101552

Umber J, Qasim M, Ashraf S et al (2023) Antioxidants mitigate oxidative stress. A general overview. In: Imran A, Hussain G (eds) The role of natural antioxidants in brain disorders. Food bioactive ingredients. Springer, Cham, pp 149–169

Victor P, Sarada D, Ramkumar KM (2021) Crosstalk between endoplasmic reticulum stress and oxidative stress: focus on protein disulfide isomerase and endoplasmic reticulum oxidase 1. Eur J Pharmacol 892:173749

Walker CL, Pomatto LCD, Tripathi DN et al (2018) Redox regulation of homeostasis and proteostasis in peroxisomes. Physiol Rev 98:89–115

Wallace DC (2013) A mitochondrial bioenergetic etiology of disease. J Clin Invest 123:1405–1412

Weinberg SE, Sena LA, Chandel NS (2015) Mitochondria in the regulation of innate and adaptive immunity. Immunity 42:406–417

Xiong YL, Guo A (2021) Animal and plant protein oxidation: chemical and functional property significance. Food Secur 10:40

Zhang R, Lei J, Chen L et al (2022) γ-Glutamylcysteine exerts neuroprotection effects against cerebral ischemia/reperfusion injury through inhibiting lipid peroxidation and ferroptosis. Antioxidants 11:1653

Part I
Biochemistry Aspects

Chapter 3
Nutritionally Mediated Oxidative Stress

3.1 Oxidative Stress at the Cellular Level

Emerging evidence indicates that a high intake of macronutrients triggers inflammation and reactive oxygen species (ROS) production by mononuclear (MNC) and polymorphonuclear (PMN) leukocytes (Tan et al. 2018). Acute ingestion of saturated fat such as cream promotes ROS production by leukocytes, which is similar in magnitude to glucose intake but more persistent and takes longer time (Dandona et al. 2010). Protein consumption also leads to an increase in oxidative ROS formation but to a much lesser extent compared to lipids and glucose (Mohanty et al. 2002). A study reported by Aljada et al. (2004) evaluated mixed meal consumption to inflammatory markers and proinflammatory cytokine production in healthy individuals. The data showed that mixed meal increased plasma C-reactive protein (CRP) levels, nuclear factor-kappa B (NF-κB) binding, and the inhibitory protein expression such as IκB kinase beta (IKK_β) and IKK_α, and p47^{phox} subunit (Aljada et al. 2004). Intakes of mixed meals also caused acute inflammatory changes with a reduction of IκBα (Aljada et al. 2004). Postprandial or nutritional or dietary oxidative stress has been used to describe the postprandial level of imbalance between the antioxidant defense and prooxidant load as a consequence of an inadequate supply of antioxidant nutrients or high oxidative load (Sies et al. 2005). The amount of caloric intake is a decisive factor influencing the intensity of postprandial oxidative stress. Overconsumption of high-calorie food leads to abnormal increases of free fatty acid (FFA), triglycerides, and blood glucose in blood circulation. High concentrations of FFA and glucose exceed the total capacity of mitochondria for oxidative phosphorylation. Ultimately, these lead to the increased transfer of single electrons to molecular oxygen. Subsequently, the superoxide anions have entered the circulation. In addition to mitochondria, ROS production by leukocytes is also influenced by the amount of caloric, in which the caloric restriction caused the decrease in protein carbonylation, lipid peroxidation, and ROS produced by leukocytes (Di Daniele et al. 2021).

In addition, the type of macronutrients consumed is also catalytic in the amplitude of postprandial oxidative stress. In lipids, the type of fat intake may play a crucial role in the immediate postprandial inflammation. Emerging evidence indicates that saturated fat is tightly linked to cardiovascular disease (CVD). While for n-3 polyunsaturated fatty acid (PUFA), Shibabaw (2021) found that PUFA exerts an anti-inflammatory effect. Despite the beneficial effect of PUFA on inflammation was reported, not all studies demonstrated such a link. Data from the human studies failed to show any benefit in postprandial plasma inflammatory cytokines after PUFA-rich meal consumption or a detrimental effect of saturated fatty acid in acute feeding (Peairs et al. 2011; Teng et al. 2014).

3.2 High Carbohydrates and Oxidative Stress

The increase in oxidative stress is associated with chronic inflammation (Wiegman et al. 2015); other sources may also further elevate the accumulation of proinflammatory cytokines in a "vicious cycle" (di Penta et al. 2013). In cultured adipocytes, ROS increases the generation of proinflammatory monocyte chemotactic protein-1 (MCP-1) and cytokine interleukin-6 (IL-6) expression (Elmarakby and Sullivan 2012; Sung et al. 2002). In adipose tissue, ROS can promote macrophage infiltration and thereby lead to a proinflammatory environment (Weisberg et al. 2003; Murphy 2009). ROS can also activate signal transduction pathways (predominantly via NF-κB), which stimulates the generation of IL-6 and tumor necrosis factor-α (TNF-α) (Park et al. 2006; Rahman et al. 2002; Elmarakby and Sullivan 2012). Moreover, oxidative stress can also stimulate cells into cellular senescence, particularly adipocyte senescence, partly through cellular oxidation damage (MacKellar et al. 2010; Minamino et al. 2009). Adipocyte senescence may recruit macrophages and promote the production of proinflammatory cytokines (Lafontan 2014; Minamino et al. 2009).

Substantial research has demonstrated that high consumption of macronutrients can promote oxidative stress, leading to inflammation through NF-κB-modulated cell signaling pathways (Tan et al. 2018). Dietary carbohydrates are particularly noteworthy, as they may contribute to long-term consequences of nutritionally mediated inflammation (Akter et al. 2022). The impact of dietary carbohydrate consumption has garnered significant attention from both academia and industry researchers due to its associations with cancer, diabetes, coronary heart disease, and obesity. High GL diets have been characterized as a common characteristic of Western culture; they are heavy in refined carbohydrates and added sugars (Clemente-Suárez et al. 2023). Conversely, low GI foods were shown to reduce postprandial glycemia in type 2 diabetes patients (Wolever et al. 2013) and obese/overweight individuals (Schwingshackl and Hoffmann 2013). Likewise, evidence from cohort and observational studies also demonstrated a relationship between high GI diets and diabetes (Dong et al. 2011; Ma et al. 2012; Bhupathiraju et al. 2014).

The high GI of white rice may contribute to high oxidative stress (Miller et al. 1992). The majority of Asian populations consume large amounts of rice as a staple food; therefore, dietary carbohydrate consumption plays a vital role in the development of metabolic ailments in Asian populations. Studies reported by Hu et al. (2012) and Nanri et al. (2010) further supported a positive relationship between total carbohydrates or rice intake and diabetes in Japanese women. Furthermore, high consumption of refined grain was also positively associated with triglyceride and fasting blood glucose levels and negatively linked to high-density lipoprotein (HDL) cholesterol in the Korean adult population and Asian Indians (Radhika et al. 2009; Song et al. 2014), imply that a high GI diet may detrimentally impact on health.

Notably, excessively high amounts of carbohydrates may result in the downregulation of transcription of insulin receptor expression and a decrease of insulin binding in the skeletal muscle (Catena et al. 2003). High glucose and insulin levels may reduce the insulin binding to insulin receptors in adipocytes (Burén et al. 2003), negatively influencing Akt activity. Decreased antioxidant capacity or accumulation of RNS/ROS due to elevated carbohydrate metabolism in insulin target tissues may alter the phosphorylation levels of these signaling pathways, and thereby lead to the deactivation. Exposure to hydrogen peroxide (H_2O_2) contributes to a significant loss in proximal and distal insulin signaling and reduced glucose transport in adipocytes and muscles *in vitro* (Henriksen et al. 2011).

Substantial evidence from epidemiological studies highlighted that refined carbohydrate intakes, for instance, fructose-rich syrups, potentially result in the epidemics of type 2 diabetes and obesity (Hu and Malik 2010; DiNicolantonio et al. 2015). Furthermore, fructose-rich syrups may also potentially pose a risk of CVD (DiNicolantonio et al. 2015). In addition to the effects mentioned above, fructose-rich diet intake may trigger metabolic and endocrine derangements, interrupting many tissues and organs in normal rats (Alzamendi et al. 2009; Francini et al. 2010). Because the liver is mainly responsible for fructose uptake and metabolism, some studies are focusing on hepatic glucose metabolism (Castro et al. 2014). Despite the molecular association underlying carbohydrate metabolism and fructose's detrimental effects requiring further elucidation, most of the experimental studies show that oxidative stress could play a crucial role (Castro et al. 2012, 2015). The key molecular mechanism to explain this association is via fructose-induced oxidative stress which subsequently results in impaired carbohydrate metabolism. The animal model study further demonstrated a greater likelihood of inflammation after feeding with fructose (Wang et al. 2020). This finding indicates the relationship between fructose and insulin resistance and its role in carbohydrate metabolism and hepatic metabolism against the anabolic pathway as well as impaired glucose tolerance (Francini et al. 2010; Castro et al. 2011, 2012). In support of this, a study reported by Castro et al. (2014) found that fructose may mediate the liver glucokinase activity through ROS production. Such findings imply that many metabolic changes triggered by fructose in the liver are more likely initiated by the elevation of fructose phosphorylation by fructokinase, followed by adaptive changes that attempt to alter the substrate flow to energy storage from mitochondrial metabolism (Castro et al. 2014).

3.3 High Animal-Based Proteins and Oxidative Stress

In developed countries, meat constitutes a significant portion of the average diet, providing 40% of daily protein, 15% of daily energy intake, and 20% of daily fat (Food and Agriculture Organization of the United Nations Statistics Division 2010). Meat is rich in saturated fatty acids (SFAs) and dietary protein. Excessive protein fermentation in the gut produces metabolites such as hydrogen sulfide (H_2S) and ammonia (NH_3), which are known to induce mucosal toxicity (Scott et al. 2013). Meat can be consumed fresh or processed through methods such as drying, stuffing, curing, fermentation, smoking, and salting (Food and Agriculture Organization of the United Nations (FAOSTAT) 2015). Despite its high protein content, meat can also be a source of mutagens. This includes polycyclic aromatic hydrocarbons (PAHs) and heterocyclic amines (HCAs) produced during grilling and high-temperature cooking, as well as N-nitroso compounds (NOCs) found in processed meats (Ledesma et al. 2016).

Intriguingly, free Fe^{2+} markedly elevates during the cooking of uncured meats. By contrast, nitrite curing prevents the degradation of heme-Fe via the stabilization of the porphyrin ring (Van Hecke et al. 2015). Heat treatment also decreases antioxidant enzymes including glutathione peroxidase (Hoac et al. 2006; Serpen et al. 2012), and produces oxygen from oxymyoglobin, which results in H_2O_2 production (Ishikawa et al. 2010). In addition, free Fe^{2+} catalyzes the Fenton reaction when oxidative processes are initiated (Bokare and Choi 2014). Through this reactive nature, ROS causes oxidative damage to meat proteins, which further explains the high formation of malondialdehyde (MDA) and 4-hydroxynonenal (4-HNE) when uncured pork is heated (Steppeler et al. 2016). Notably, a study found a relatively low concentration of simple aldehydes in overcooked uncured pork compared to cooked meat. This finding could be attributed to the evaporation of aldehydes caused by the decrease of the prooxidant effect of oxymyoglobin when intense heating or heated to above 75 °C (Bou et al. 2008). When the meats are nitrite-cured, less degradation of the heat-stable NO-heme may cause a decreased release of Fe^{2+} to initiate oxidation processes, thereby leading to the reduction of lipid oxidation. Fenton reaction is a chain reaction and thus a higher concentration of oxidation products after digestion was expected (Van Hecke et al. 2014). A study reported by Van Hecke et al. (2015) revealed that the antioxidant effect of nitrite-curing during digestion was significantly decreased in overcooked nitrite-cured pork. In support of this, a temperature reaching 80 °C or a prolonged cooking time elevated the decomposition of nitrite (Okayama et al. 1991). A 1: 1 ratio of nitric oxide ('NO) to ROS promotes lipid oxidation, while 'NO > ROS inhibits this process (Darley-Usmar et al. 1995). Accordingly, low residual nitrite contributed by intense heating is more likely to modify the •NO: ROS ratio; therefore, nitrite could convert to pro-oxidant behavior from an antioxidant, which may explain the elevated formation of oxidation products in overcooked nitrite-cured meats. MDA was demonstrated to be absorbed in the bloodstream and generate lipid oxidation products that could reach tissues and result in DNA damage (Ayala et al. 2014). Indeed, low lipid oxidation products in colonic digests are due to Schiff base formation with proteins, and thereby interact with bacterial DNA (Nair et al. 2007) or are oxidized by bacterial aldehyde dehydrogenase activity. Taken together, the effect of nitrite curing of meat in the colonic step was predominant since it was associated with a low amount of MDA but proportionally elevated 4-HNE levels and doubled heptanal levels in the cooked and overcooked meats (Van Hecke et al. 2015).

Furthermore, the nitrite-curing of pork and beef also contributed to a two-fold difference in heptanal levels in activated colonic digests compared to their counterparts (Van Hecke et al. 2014). Lipid aldehydes, for instance, MDA and 4-HNE, bind with protein chains causing the protein to be less susceptible to pepsin activity and leading to protein aggregation (Van Hecke et al. 2014). Overcooked nitrite-cured pork demonstrated a low dosage of lipid oxidation products and protein carbonyl compounds before digestion; this is more likely to occur because the meat protein is initially well-digested in the stomach, after which the low amount of residual protein reacts with MDA and 4-HNE, and thus form in a later phase of digestion (Van Hecke et al. 2014). The rate of protein digestibility is crucial in association with colorectal cancer because higher amounts of residual protein reaching the colon could lead to the formation of potentially harmful protein fermentation products, for instance, indole, p-cresol, phenol, and ammonia (Windey et al. 2012). NOC can be activated either nonenzymatically or enzymatically via oxidation (Tsutsumi et al. 2010; Miura et al. 2011). The nonenzymatic activation of NOC can be produced by a hydroxyl radical-generating system comprised of Fe^{2+}, H_2O_2, ascorbic acid, and Cu^{2+}. All these compounds are often present in meat. When Cu^{2+}, Fe^{2+}, or H_2O_2 was eliminated from a reaction mixture with N-nitroso-N-methylpentylamine, the mutagenicity of these compounds was decreased (Miura et al. 2011).

3.4   Excessive Consumption of Fats and Oxidative Stress

Evidence from systematic reviews of prospective cohort studies (Siri-Tarino et al. 2010; Chowdhury et al. 2014) and randomized trials (Chowdhury et al. 2014; Harcombe et al. 2015) has called for a reevaluation of dietary guidelines regarding saturated fatty acid (SFA) intake and a reassessment of their impact on health. While many studies have linked SFAs to cardiovascular disease (CVD) (Maki et al. 2021), not all research supports this association (Valk et al. 2022). For instance, a study by De Souza et al. (2015) found no association between SFA consumption and ischemic stroke, CVD, type 2 diabetes, or coronary heart disease. Interestingly, other research has shown that types of fat and total fat intake were negatively associated with total mortality (Dehghan et al. 2017). Furthermore, no relationship was found between types of fat or total fat intake and myocardial infarction or CVD mortality (Dehghan et al. 2017).

Notably, SFAs including palmitic acid and lauric acid, did not activate Toll-like receptors 2 (TLR2) or 4 (TLR4) in HEK-Blue cells transfected with these receptors (Murumalla and Gunasekaran 2012). Although some research indicates an inverse association between TLR2 or TLR4 activation and SFAs, not all studies support this link. For example, Huang et al. (2012) found that lauric acid and palmitic acid stimulated TLR4 and TLR2 in transiently transfected human monocytic (THP-1) monocytes and RAW264.7 macrophages. Despite the limited evidence on the impact of SFAs on gene expression, epidemiological studies have reported associations between SFA intake and CVD. However, meta-analyses of prospective studies generally show a weak association between SFAs and CVD risk. Evidence from randomized trials indicates that substituting polyunsaturated fatty acids (PUFAs) for SFAs does not significantly alter CVD risk (Hoenselaar 2012). Inconclusive research suggests that SFAs, despite their general classification, might have potential health benefits. For instance, medium-chain SFAs could help suppress body fat accumulation and prevent obesity (Nagao and Yanagita 2010). Additionally, Youseef-Elabd et al. (2012) investigated the impact of a high-SFA diet on gene expression in adipose tissue. Their study found that an SFA-rich diet led to the upregulation of transcriptional factors such as cathepsin S (*CTSS*), interleukin-8 (*IL-8*), and integrin beta 2 (*ITGB2*), particularly in moderately overweight individuals. These findings suggest that the observed changes in gene expression were associated with diet-induced effects rather than obesity itself.

A high-fat diet (HFD) was shown to be a significant risk factor for health. The data from the animal model studies showed that feeding animals with an HFD in the long-term promotes dysfunctional mitochondria in some organs and increases oxidative stress (Bruce et al. 2009; Yokota et al. 2009; Ballal et al. 2010). Substantial studies indicate that high-fat intakes lead to a significant reduction in auditory function (Gopinath et al. 2011; Spankovich et al. 2011). The data showed that long-term HFD caused age-related hearing loss and decreased auditory function (Du et al. 2012). From the study reviewed, feeding rats with an HFD for 12 months may elevate total cholesterol, plasma triglycerides, and nonesterified fatty acid levels, leading to an increase in blood oxidative stress parameters. In addition to the effects observed in the lipid profile, HFD also induced mitochondrial damage and increased ROS accumulation in the inner ear (Du et al. 2012), indicating enormous detrimental impacts of an HFD on health.

In support of this, some research has found that obesity or increased caloric intake is linked to an elevation of mitochondrial superoxide production. Feeding both mice and humans with an HFD results in a significant increase in H_2O_2 production from the mitochondria isolated from the skeletal muscle (Anderson et al. 2009). Moreover, accumulation of ROS has also been found in mitochondria isolated from the liver (Raffaella et al. 2008), adipose (Curtis et al. 2010), and kidney (Ruggiero et al. 2011) tissues in obese-treated or high-fat animals. Valenzuela et al. (2017) further revealed that feeding with an HFD diet significantly decreased liver enzyme activity, for instance, glutathione peroxidase, superoxide dismutase (SOD), glutathione reductase, and catalase in mice.

The accumulation of adipose tissue and an adipogenic diet can induce oxidative stress in mammalian tissues. Several studies have emerged to support the hypothesis that HFD enhances inflammation in the intestine, for instance, the small intestine. This finding may represent an early event that predisposes and precedes the individual to obesity and insulin resistance (Sun et al. 2016). The animal model further demonstrated that feeding obesity-prone Sprague-Dawley rats with HFD stimulates myeloperoxidase activity, an inflammation marker, in the ileum (de La Serre et al. 2010). In support of this, an animal study has further demonstrated that feeding the HFD diet stimulates macrophage migration inhibitory factor expression in the ileum of obesity-prone C57BL/6 J mice (de Wit et al. 2008). Several studies have also reached a similar finding, in which administration of HFD after 2 to 6 weeks activated TNF-α expression and increased body fat mass and weight gain (Ding et al. 2010; Cortez et al. 2013). Furthermore, high-fat intakes also increase the M1-polarized population and activate Kupffer cells (the resident macrophages of the liver) in mice, which is associated with insulin resistance and pathogenesis of obesity-induced fatty liver disease (Gao et al. 2010). In this regard, obesity is linked to a marked elevation of oxidative damage to all cellular macromolecules (Grimsrud et al. 2007, 2008; Matsuda and Shimomura 2013).

The mode of action underlying the increase of oxidative stress in metabolic ailments is not fully understood, but it is hypothesized that mitochondrial dysfunction (Yuzefovych et al. 2013), aggravated by NADPH oxidase activity (Furukawa et al. 2004), and elevated fatty acid oxidation (Lee et al. 2015) contribute to this phenomenon. Most of the studies highlighted abnormal gene expression in the liver and adipose tissues, accompanied by downregulation of antioxidative enzyme expression and increased NADPH oxidase levels (Lee 2013; Le Lay et al. 2014). HFD promotes dyslipidemia, which is linked to oxidative stress, an elevation of free radicals, and the accumulation of several transition metals (Charradi et al. 2013). Furthermore, fat accumulation has also been associated with systemic oxidative stress in humans and mice via accumulation of ROS (Le Lay et al. 2014). HFD promotes oxidative stress and lipid peroxidation, whereas NADPH oxidase stimulation decreases the generation of redox-sensitive transcription mRNA, for instance, NF-κB and adipocytokines (fat-derived hormones) such as adiponectin, monocyte chemotactic protein-1 (MCP-1), IL-6, plasminogen activator inhibitor-1, and other inflammatory cytokines from various metabolic tissues (Kaur 2014).

Moreover, HFD increases the chylomicrons level in the intestine. The chylomicrons enter the bloodstream and lead to the production of free fatty acids (FFAs), which are taken up by the liver. The hepatic FFAs may either be esterified into triglycerides or enter the mitochondria for β-oxidation (Pessayre et al. 2001; Cole et al. 2011). Triglycerides either produce very low-density lipoprotein (VLDL) or accumulate in hepatocytes as small droplets and thereby shift into low-density lipoprotein (LDL) (Pessayre et al. 2001). High LDL burden in the blood due to lack of or excessive accumulation of LDL-receptors in hepatocytes may form oxidized LDL (Ox-LDL), which is subsequently engulfed by macrophages to become foam cells. Accordingly, foam cells accumulate in the arterial endothelium to form plaque. Lastly, these lead to circulatory and cardiovascular disorders including atherosclerosis, thromboembolism, heart block, and hypertension (Horton et al. 2002; Mitra et al. 2011; Pirillo et al. 2013). The mitochondrial β-oxidation of FFAs is associated with the conversion into reduced cofactors $FADH_2$ and NADH from oxidized cofactors (FAD and NAD^+), which in turn reoxidized and restored into FAD and NAD^+ via the mitochondrial respiratory chain. $FADH_2$ and NADH transfer electrons to the first complexes of the respiratory chain during reoxidation. Most of the electrons are migrated up to cytochrome-c oxidase and subsequently form water by combining with oxygen and protons. These intermediates may bind with oxygen and generate more and more superoxide anion radicals and other ROS (Pessayre et al. 2002; Matsuzawa-Nagata et al. 2008; Hamanaka and Chandel 2010; Brand 2010). Hence, excessive consumption of fat-rich diets triggers mitochondrial β-oxidation of FFAs and thereby results in an excess electron flow using cytochrome-c oxidase, which increases the accumulation of ROS. Mitochondria are a crucial cellular source of ROS; they oxidize the unsaturated lipids of fat deposits to result in lipid peroxidation. Lipid peroxidation and ROS can consume antioxidant enzymes and vitamins (Pessayre et al. 2002; Jain and Micinski 2013). Reduction of these protective substances may prevent ROS inactivation and cause lipid peroxidation and ROS-mediated damage (Le Lay et al. 2014). This HFD-induced ROS may activate the proinflammatory level and subsequently stimulate the NF-κB transcription factor. In addition, HFD may also induce NF-κB or ROS, which triggers NF-κB-dependent proinflammatory agents, for instance, inducible nitric oxide synthase (iNOS), interferon-γ (IFN-γ), and tumor necrosis factor alpha (TNF-α) (Weisberg et al. 2008; Ruggiero et al. 2011; Vial et al. 2011). Such findings highlight the role of oxidative stress triggered by HFD in metabolic ailments. Intriguingly, an *in vitro* study demonstrated that free fatty acids promote ROS accumulation, suggesting that elevated fatty acids in obesity may provide an extra source of additional electron transport chain substrates through fatty acid oxidation (Furukawa et al. 2004; Kawasaki et al. 2012). Besides ROS production, the excessive generation of nitric oxide (NO) via the stimulation of iNOS also leads to an accumulation of RNS (Rahman et al. 2001; Savini et al. 2013).

Collectively, chronic intakes of high glycemic index foods may result in oxidative stress through the formation of free radicals that are capable of damaging biological molecules and promoting abnormal cell proliferation via gene mutation (Brownlee 2005). Moreover, HCA produced during grilling and high-temperature cooking of meat may lead to the oxidation of lipids and proteins, and subsequently cause oxidative stress and thereby increase the risk of chronic diseases (Carvalho et al. 2015). The HFD may act as a stimulus to increase the systemic inflammatory response in the development of diabetes, obesity, cancers, and CVD (Grivennikov et al. 2010; Wijnstok et al. 2010; Fedele et al. 2011; Grange et al. 2011). Taken together, these findings suggest that high-calorie/high-carbohydrate/high-fat diets activate oxidative stress by increasing inflammatory markers and augmenting the inflammatory response.

References

Akter S, Akhter H, Chaudhury HS et al (2022) Dietary carbohydrates: pathogenesis and potential therapeutic targets to obesity-associated metabolic syndrome. Biofactors 48:1036–1059

Aljada A, Mohanty P, Ghanim H et al (2004) Increase in intranuclear nuclear factor kappaB and decrease in inhibitor kappaB in mononuclear cells after a mixed meal: evidence for a proinflammatory effect. Am J Clin Nutr 79:682–690

Alzamendi A, Giovambattista A, Raschia A et al (2009) Fructose-rich diet-induced abdominal adipose tissue endocrine dysfunction in normal male rats. Endocrine 35:227–232

Anderson EJ, Lustig ME, Boyle KE et al (2009) Mitochondrial H_2O_2 emission and cellular redox state link excess fat intake to insulin resistance in both rodents and humans. J Clin Invest 119:573–581

Ayala A, Muñoz MF, Argüelles S (2014) Lipid peroxidation: production, metabolism, and signaling mechanisms of malondialdehyde and 4-hydroxy-2-nonenal. Oxid Med Cell Longev., Article ID 360438:31

Ballal K, Wilson CR, Harmancey R et al (2010) Obesogenic high fat western diet induces oxidative stress and apoptosis in rat heart. Mol Cell Biochem 344:221–230

Bhupathiraju SN, Tobias DK, Malik VS et al (2014) Glycemic index, glycemic load, and risk of type 2 diabetes: results from 3 large US cohorts and an updated meta-analysis. Am J Clin Nutr 100:218–232

Bokare AD, Choi W (2014) Review of iron-free Fenton-like systems for activating H_2O_2 in advanced oxidation processes. J Hazard Mater 275:121–135

Bou R, Guardiola F, Codony R et al (2008) Effect of heating oxymyoglobin and metmyoglobin on the oxidation of muscle microsomes. J Agric Food Chem 56:9612–9620

Brand MD (2010) The sites and topology of mitochondrial superoxide production. Exp Gerontol 45:466–472

Brownlee M (2005) The pathobiology of diabetic complications: a unifying mechanism. Diabetes 54:1615–1625

Bruce KD, Cagampang FR, Argenton M et al (2009) Maternal high-fat feeding primes steatohepatitis in adult mice offspring, involving mitochondrial dysfunction and altered lipogenesis gene expression. Hepatology 50:1796–1808

Burén J, Liu H-X, Lauritz J et al (2003) High glucose and insulin in combination cause insulin receptor substrate-1 and -2 depletion and protein kinase B desensitisation in primary cultured rat adipocytes: possible implications for insulin resistance in type 2 diabetes. Eur J Endocrinol 148:157–167

Carvalho AM, Miranda AM, Santos FA et al (2015) High intake of heterocyclic amines from meat is associated with oxidative stress. Br J Nutr 113:1301–1307

Castro MC, Massa ML, Del Zotto H (2011) Rat liver uncoupling protein 2: changes induced by a fructose-rich diet. Life Sci 89:609–614

Castro MC, Francini F, Schinella G et al (2012) Apocynin administration prevents the changes induced by a fructose-rich diet on rat liver metabolism and the antioxidant system. Clin Sci 123:681–692

Castro MC, Francini F, Gagliardino JJ et al (2014) Lipoic acid prevents fructose-induced changes in liver carbohydrate metabolism: role of oxidative stress. Biochim Biophys Acta 1840:1145–1151

Castro MC, Massa ML, Arbeláez LG et al (2015) Fructose-induced inflammation, insulin resistance and oxidative stress: a liver pathological triad effectively disrupted by lipoic acid. Life Sci 137:1–6

Catena C, Cavarape A, Novello M et al (2003) Insulin receptors and renal sodium handling in hypertensive fructose-fed rats. Kidney Int 64:2163–2171

Charradi K, Elkahoui S, Limam F et al (2013) High-fat diet induced an oxidative stress in white adipose tissue and disturbed plasma transition metals in rat: prevention by grape seed and skin extract. J Physiol Sci 63:445–455

Chowdhury R, Warnakula S, Kunutsor S et al (2014) Association of dietary, circulating, and sup-
plement fatty acids with coronary risk: a systematic review and meta-analysis. Ann Intern Med
160:398–406

Clemente-Suárez VJ, Beltrán-Velasco AI, Redondo-Flórez L et al (2023) Global impacts of
Western diet and its effects on metabolism and health: a narrative review. Nutrients 15:2749

Cole MA, Murray AJ, Cochlin LE et al (2011) A high fat diet increases mitochondrial fatty acid
oxidation and uncoupling to decrease efficiency in rat heart. Basic Res Cardiol 106:447–457

Cortez M, Carmo LS, Rogero MM et al (2013) A high-fat diet increases IL-1, IL-6, and TNF-α
production by increasing NF-κB and attenuating PPAR-γ expression in bone marrow mesen-
chymal stem cells. Inflammation 36:379–386

Curtis JM, Grimsrud PA, Wright WS et al (2010) Downregulation of adipose glutathione
S-transferase A4 leads to increased protein carbonylation, oxidative stress, and mitochondrial
dysfunction. Diabetes 59:1132–1142

Dandona P, Ghanim H, Chaudhuri A et al (2010) Macronutrient intake induces oxidative and
inflammatory stress: potential relevance to atherosclerosis and insulin resistance. Exp Mol Med
42:245–253

Darley-Usmar V, Wiseman H, Halliwell B (1995) Nitric oxide and oxygen radicals: a question of
balance. FEBS Lett 369:131–135

de La Serre CB, Ellis CL, Lee J et al (2010) Propensity to high-fat diet-induced obesity in rats is
associated with changes in the gut microbiota and gut inflammation. Am J Physiol Gastrointest
Liver Physiol 299:G440–G448

De Souza RJ, Mente A, Maroleanu A et al (2015) Intake of saturated and trans unsaturated fatty
acids and risk of all cause mortality, cardiovascular disease, and type 2 diabetes: systematic
review and meta-analysis of observational studies. BMJ 351:h3978

de Wit NJ, Bosch-Vermeulen H, de Groot PJ et al (2008) The role of the small intestine in the
development of dietary fat-induced obesity and insulin resistance in C57BL/6J mice. BMC
Med Genet 1:14

Dehghan M, Mente A, Zhang X et al (2017) Associations of fats and carbohydrate intake with cardiovascular disease and mortality in 18 countries from five continents (PURE): a prospective
cohort study. Lancet 390:2050–2062

Di Daniele N, Marrone G, Di Lauro M et al (2021) Effects of caloric restriction diet on arterial
hypertension and endothelial dysfunction. Nutrients 13:274

di Penta A, Moreno B, Reix S et al (2013) Oxidative stress and proinflammatory cytokines contribute to demyelination and axonal damage in a cerebellar culture model of neuroinflammation.
PLoS One 8:e54722

Ding S, Chi MM, Scull BP et al (2010) High-fat diet: bacteria interactions promote intestinal
inflammation which precedes and correlates with obesity and insulin resistance in mouse.
PLoS One 5:e12191

DiNicolantonio JJ, O'Keefe JH, Lucan SC (2015) Added fructose: a principle driver of type 2
diabetes mellitus and its consequences. Mayo Clin Proc 90:372–381

Dong JY, Zhang L, Zhang YH et al (2011) Dietary glycaemic index and glycaemic load in relation to the risk of type 2 diabetes: a meta-analysis of prospective cohort studies. Br J Nutr
106:1649–1654

Du Z, Yang Y, Hu Y et al (2012) A long-term high-fat diet increases oxidative stress, mitochondrial
damage and apoptosis in the inner ear of D-galactose-induced aging rats. Hear Res 287:15–24

Elmarakby AA, Sullivan JC (2012) Relationship between oxidative stress and inflammatory cytokines in diabetic nephropathy. Cardiovasc Ther 30:49–59

Fedele S, Sabbah W, Donos N et al (2011) Common oral mucosal diseases, systemic inflammation,
and cardiovascular diseases in a large cross-sectional US survey. Am Heart J 161:344–350

Food and Agriculture Organization of the United Nations (FAOSTAT) (2015). http://faostat3.fao.
org/download/Q/QL/E

Food and Agriculture Organization of the United Nations Statistics Division (2010) Food balance sheets millennium issue 1999–2001 special charts. http://www.fao.org/economic/ess/food-balance-sheets-millennium-issue-1999-2001-special-charts/en/

Francini F, Castro MC, Schinella G et al (2010) Changes induced by a fructose-rich diet on hepatic metabolism and the antioxidant system. Life Sci 86:965–971

Furukawa S, Fujita T, Shimabukuro M et al (2004) Increased oxidative stress in obesity and its impact on metabolic syndrome. J Clin Invest 114:1752–1761

Gao D, Nong S, Huang X et al (2010) The effects of palmitate on hepatic insulin resistance are mediated by NADPH oxidase 3-derived reactive oxygen species through JNK and p38MAPK pathways. J Biol Chem 285:29965–29973

Gopinath B, Flood VM, Teber E et al (2011) Dietary intake of cholesterol is positively associated and use of cholesterol-lowering medication is negatively associated with prevalent age-related hearing loss. J Nutr 141:1355–1361

Grange JM, Krone B, Mastrangelo G (2011) Infection, inflammation and cancer. Int J Cancer 128:2240–2241

Grimsrud PA, Picklo MJ, Griffin TJ et al (2007) Carbonylation of adipose proteins in obesity and insulin resistance: identification of adipocyte fatty acid-binding protein as a cellular target of 4-hydroxynonenal. Mol Cell Proteomics 6:624–637

Grimsrud PA, Xie H, Griffin TJ et al (2008) Oxidative stress and covalent modification of protein with bioactive aldehydes. J Biol Chem 283:21837–21841

Grivennikov SI, Greten FR, Karin M (2010) Immunity, inflammation, and cancer. Cell 140:883–899

Hamanaka RB, Chandel NS (2010) Mitochondrial reactive oxygen species regulate cellular signaling and dictate biological outcomes. Trends Biochem Sci 35:505–513

Harcombe Z, Baker JS, Cooper SM et al (2015) Evidence from randomised controlled trials did not support the introduction of dietary fat guidelines in 1977 and 1983: a systematic review and meta-analysis. Open Heart 2:e000196

Henriksen EJ, Diamond-Stanic MK, Marchionne EM (2011) Oxidative stress and the etiology of insulin resistance and type 2 diabetes. Free Radic Biol Med 51:993–999

Hoac T, Daun C, Trafikowska U et al (2006) Influence of heat treatment on lipid oxidation and glutathione peroxidase activity in chicken and duck meat. Innovative Food Sci. Emerg. Technol. 7:88–93

Hoenselaar R (2012) Saturated fat and cardiovascular disease: the discrepancy between the scientific literature and dietary advice. Nutrition 28:118–123

Horton JD, Goldstein JL, Brown MS (2002) SREBPs: activators of the complete program of cholesterol and fatty acid synthesis in the liver. J Clin Invest 109:1125–1131

Hu FB, Malik VS (2010) Sugar-sweetened beverages and risk of obesity and type 2 diabetes: epidemiologic evidence. Physiol Behav 100:47–54

Hu EA, Pan A, Malik V et al (2012) White rice consumption and risk of type 2 diabetes: meta-analysis and systematic review. BMJ 344:e1454

Huang S, Rutkowsky JM, Snodgrass RG et al (2012) Saturated fatty acids activate TLR-mediated proinflammatory signaling pathways. J Lipid Res 53:2002–2013

Ishikawa S, Tamaki S, Ohata M et al (2010) Heme induces DNA damage and hyperproliferation of colonic epithelial cells via hydrogen peroxide produced by heme oxygenase: a possible mechanism of heme-induced colon cancer. Mol Nutr Food Res 54:1182–1191

Jain SK, Micinski D (2013) Vitamin D upregulates glutamate cysteine ligase and glutathione reductase, and GSH formation, and decreases ROS and MCP-1 and IL-8 secretion in high-glucose exposed U937 monocytes. Biochem Biophys Res Commun 437:7–11

Kaur J (2014) A comprehensive review on metabolic syndrome. Cardiol Res Practice 2014., Article ID 943162:21

Kawasaki N, Asada R, Saito A et al (2012) Obesity-induced endoplasmic reticulum stress causes chronic inflammation in adipose tissue. Sci Rep 2:799

Lafontan M (2014) Adipose tissue and adipocyte dysregulation. Diabetes Metab 40:16–28

Le Lay S, Simard G, Martinez MC et al (2014) Oxidative stress and metabolic pathologies: from an adipocentric point of view. Oxid Med Cell Longev., Article ID 908539:18

Ledesma E, Rendueles M, Díaz M (2016) Contamination of meat products during smoking by polycyclic aromatic hydrocarbons: processes and prevention. Food Control 60:64–87

Lee CY (2013) The effect of high-fat diet-induced pathophysiological changes in the gut on obesity: what should be the ideal treatment? Clin. Transl. Gastroenterol. 4:e39

Lee J, Ellis JM, Wolfgang MJ (2015) Adipose fatty acid oxidation is required for thermogenesis and potentiates oxidative stress-induced inflammation. Cell Rep 10:266–279

Ma XY, Liu JP, Song ZY (2012) Glycemic load, glycemic index and risk of cardiovascular diseases: meta-analyses of prospective studies. Atherosclerosis 223:491–496

MacKellar J, Cushman SW, Periwal V (2010) Waves of adipose tissue growth in the genetically obese Zucker fatty rat. PLoS One 5:e8197

Maki KC, Dicklin MR, Kirkpatrick CF (2021) Saturated fats and cardiovascular health: current evidence and controversies. J Clin Lipidol 15:765–772

Matsuda M, Shimomura I (2013) Increased oxidative stress in obesity: implications for metabolic syndrome, diabetes, hypertension, dyslipidemia, atherosclerosis, and cancer. Obes. Res. Clin. Pract. 7:e330–e341

Matsuzawa-Nagata N, Takamura T, Ando H et al (2008) Increased oxidative stress precedes the onset of high-fat diet-induced insulin resistance and obesity. Metabolism 57:1071–1077

Miller JB, Pang E, Bramall L (1992) Rice: a high or low glycemic index food? Am J Clin Nutr 56:1034–1036

Minamino T, Orimo M, Shimizu I et al (2009) A crucial role for adipose tissue p53 in the regulation of insulin resistance. Nat Med 15:1082–1087

Mitra S, Goyal T, Mehta JL (2011) Oxidized LDL, LOX-1 and atherosclerosis. Cardiovasc Drugs Ther 25:419–429

Miura M, Inami K, Yoshida M et al (2011) Isolation and structural identification of a direct-acting mutagen derived from N-nitroso-N-methylpentylamine and Fenton's reagent with copper ion. Bioorg Med Chem 19:5693–5697

Mohanty P, Ghanim H, Hamouda W et al (2002) Both lipid and protein intakes stimulate increased generation of reactive oxygen species by polymorphonuclear leukocytes and mononuclear cells. Am J Clin Nutr 75:767–772

Murphy MP (2009) How mitochondria produce reactive oxygen species. Biochem J 417:1–13

Murumalla RK, Gunasekaran MK (2012) Fatty acids do not pay the toll: effect of SFA and PUFA on human adipose tissue and mature adipocytes inflammation. Lipids Health Dis 11:175

Nagao K, Yanagita T (2010) Medium-chain fatty acids: functional lipids for the prevention and treatment of the metabolic syndrome. Pharmacol Res 61:208–212

Nair U, Bartsch H, Nair J (2007) Lipid peroxidation-induced DNA damage in cancer-prone inflammatory diseases: a review of published adduct types and levels in humans. Free Radic Biol Med 43:1109–1120

Nanri A, Mizoue T, Noda M et al (2010) Rice intake and type 2 diabetes in Japanese men and women: the Japan public health center-based prospective study. Am J Clin Nutr 92:1468–1477

Okayama T, Fujii M, Yamanoue M (1991) Effect of cooking temperature on the percentage colour formation, nitrite decomposition and sarcoplasmic protein denaturation in processed meat products. Meat Sci 30:49–57

Park J, Choe SS, Choi AH et al (2006) Increase in glucose-6-phosphate dehydrogenase in adipocytes stimulates oxidative stress and inflammatory signals. Diabetes 55:2939–2949

Peairs AD, Rankin JW, Lee YW (2011) Effects of acute ingestion of different fats on oxidative stress and inflammation in overweight and obese adults. Nutr J 10:122

Pessayre D, Berson A, Fromenty B et al (2001) Mitochondria in steatohepatitis. Semin Liver Dis 21:057–070

Pessayre D, Mansouri A, Fromenty B (2002) Nonalcoholic steatosis and steatohepatitis. V. Mitochondrial dysfunction in steatohepatitis. Am. J. Physiol. Gastrointest. Liver Physiol. 282:G193–G199

Pirillo A, Norata GD, Catapano AL (2013) LOX-1, OxLDL, and atherosclerosis. Mediat Inflamm., Article ID 152786:12

Radhika G, Van Dam RM, Sudha V et al (2009) Refined grain consumption and the metabolic syndrome in urban Asian Indians (Chennai urban rural epidemiology study 57). Metabolism 58:675–681

Raffaella C, Francesca B, Italia F et al (2008) Alterations in hepatic mitochondrial compartment in a model of obesity and insulin resistance. Obesity 16:958–964

Rahman MM, Varghese Z, Moorhead JF (2001) Paradoxical increase in nitric oxide synthase activity in hypercholesterolaemic rats with impaired renal function and decreased activity of nitric oxide. Nephrol. Dial. Transplant. 16:262–268

Rahman I, Gilmour PS, Jimenez LA et al (2002) Oxidative stress and TNF-α induce histone acetylation and NF-κB/AP-1 activation in alveolar epithelial cells: potential mechanism in gene transcription in lung inflammation. Mol Cell Biochem 234(235):239–248

Ruggiero C, Ehrenshaft M, Cleland E et al (2011) High-fat diet induces an initial adaptation of mitochondrial bioenergetics in the kidney despite evident oxidative stress and mitochondrial ROS production. Am J Physiol Endocrinol Metab 300:E1047–E1058

Savini I, Catani MV, Evangelista D et al (2013) Obesity-associated oxidative stress: strategies finalized to improve redox state. Int J Mol Sci 14:10497–10538

Schwingshackl L, Hoffmann G (2013) Long-term effects of low glycemic index/load vs. high glycemic index/load diets on parameters of obesity and obesity-associated risks: a systematic review and meta-analysis. Nutr Metab Cardiovasc Dis 23:699–706

Scott KP, Gratz SW, Sheridan PO et al (2013) The influence of diet on the gut microbiota. Pharmacol Res 69:52–60

Serpen A, Gökmen V, Fogliano V (2012) Total antioxidant capacities of raw and cooked meats. Meat Sci 90:60–65

Shibabaw T (2021) Omega-3 polyunsaturated fatty acids: anti-inflammatory and anti-hypertriglyceridemia mechanisms in cardiovascular disease. Mol Cell Biochem 476:993–1003

Sies H, Stahl W, Sevanian A (2005) Nutritional, dietary and postprandial oxidative stress. J Nutr 135:969–972

Siri-Tarino PW, Sun Q, Hu FB et al (2010) Meta-analysis of prospective cohort studies evaluating the association of saturated fat with cardiovascular disease. Am J Clin Nutr 91:535–546

Song S, Lee JE, Song WO et al (2014) Carbohydrate intake and refined-grain consumption are associated with metabolic syndrome in the Korean adult population. J Acad Nutr Diet 114:54–62

Spankovich C, Hood LJ, Silver HJ et al (2011) Associations between diet and both high and low pure tone averages and transient evoked otoacoustic emissions in an older adult population-based study. J Am Acad Audiol 22:49–58

Steppeler C, Haugen J-E, Rødbotten R et al (2016) Formation of malondialdehyde, 4-hydroxynonenal, and 4-hydroxyhexenal during in vitro digestion of cooked beef, pork, chicken, and salmon. J Agric Food Chem 64:487–496

Sun J, Qiao Y, Qi C et al (2016) High-fat-diet–induced obesity is associated with decreased anti-inflammatory Lactobacillus reuteri sensitive to oxidative stress in mouse Peyer's patches. Nutrition 32:265–272

Sung FL, Zhu TY, Au-Yeung KKW et al (2002) Enhanced MCP-1 expression during ischemia/reperfusion injury is mediated by oxidative stress and NF-κB. Kidney Int 62:1160–1170

Tan BL, Norhaizan ME, Liew W-P-P (2018) Nutrients and oxidative stress: friend or foe? Oxid Med Cell Longev., Article ID 9719584:24

Teng KT, Chang CY, Chang LF et al (2014) Modulation of obesity-induced inflammation by dietary fats: mechanisms and clinical evidence. Nutr J 13:12

Tsutsumi N, Inami K, Mochizuki M (2010) Activation mechanism for N-nitroso-N-methylbutylamine mutagenicity by radical species. Bioorg Med Chem 18:8284–8288

Valenzuela R, Echeverria F, Ortiz M et al (2017) Hydroxytyrosol prevents reduction in liver activity of Δ-5 and Δ-6 desaturases, oxidative stress, and depletion in long chain polyunsaturated fatty acid content in different tissues of high-fat diet fed mice. Lipids Health Dis 16:64

Valk R, Hammill J, Grip J (2022) Saturated fat: villain and bogeyman in the development of cardiovascular disease? Eur J Prev Cardiol 29:2312–2321

Van Hecke T, Vanden Bussche J, Vanhaecke L et al (2014) Nitrite curing of chicken, pork, and beef inhibits oxidation but does not affect N-nitroso compound (NOC)-specific DNA adduct formation during in vitro digestion. J Agric Food Chem 62:1980–1988

Van Hecke T, Vossen E, Hemeryck LY et al (2015) Increased oxidative and nitrosative reactions during digestion could contribute to the association between well-done red meat consumption and colorectal cancer. Food Chem 187:29–36

Vial G, Dubouchaud H, Couturier K et al (2011) Effects of a high-fat diet on energy metabolism and ROS production in rat liver. J Hepatol 54:348–356

Wang Y, Qi W, Song G et al (2020) High-fructose diet increases inflammatory cytokines and alters gut microbiota composition in rats. Mediators Inflam., Article ID 6672636:10

Weisberg SP, McCann D, Desai M et al (2003) Obesity is associated with macrophage accumulation in adipose tissue. J Clin Invest 112:1796–1808

Weisberg SP, Leibel R, Tortoriello DV (2008) Dietary curcumin significantly improves obesity-associated inflammation and diabetes in mouse models of diabesity. Endocrinology 149:3549–3558

Wiegman CH, Michaeloudes C, Haji G et al (2015) Oxidative stress–induced mitochondrial dysfunction drives inflammation and airway smooth muscle remodeling in patients with chronic obstructive pulmonary disease. J Allergy Clin Immunol 136:769–780

Wijnstok NJ, Twisk JW, Young IS et al (2010) Inflammation markers are associated with cardiovascular diseases risk in adolescents: the Young hearts project 2000. J Adolesc Health 47:346–351

Windey K, De Preter V, Verbeke K (2012) Relevance of protein fermentation to gut health. Mol Nutr Food Res 56:184–196

Wolever TM, Gibbs AL, Chiasson JL et al (2013) Altering source or amount of dietary carbohydrate has acute and chronic effects on postprandial glucose and triglycerides in type 2 diabetes: Canadian trial of carbohydrates in diabetes (CCD). Nutr Metab Cardiovasc Dis 23:227–234

Yokota T, Kinugawa S, Hirabayashi K et al (2009) Oxidative stress in skeletal muscle impairs mitochondrial respiration and limits exercise capacity in type 2 diabetic mice. Am J Physiol Heart Circ Physiol 297:H1069–H1077

Youseef-Elabd EM, McGee KC, Tripathi G et al (2012) Acute and chronic saturated fatty acid treatment as a key investigator of the TLR-mediated inflammatory response in human adipose tissue, in vitro. J Nutr Biochem 23:39–50

Yuzefovych LV, Musiyenko SI, Wilson GL et al (2013) Mitochondrial DNA damage and dysfunction, and oxidative stress are associated with endoplasmic reticulum stress, protein degradation and apoptosis in high fat diet-induced insulin resistance mice. PLoS One 8:e54059

Chapter 4
Molecular Mechanisms of Oxidative Stress-Induced Diseases

Emerging research evidence has suggested that low-grade chronic systemic inflammation plays a vitally important role in modulating several chronic diseases such as cancer, cardiovascular disease (CVD), metabolic syndrome, and type 2 diabetes (Tan et al. 2018a, b), which is known as "inflammatory diseases" (Su and Peng 2020). Although the underlying molecular inflammatory process involved in each disease may vary from other diseases, the basic mode of action of the inflammatory mediators and proinflammatory cytokines are similar (Zhao et al. 2023). The molecular connectivity of oxidative stress-induced diseases will be described in the following section.

4.1 Obesity and Adipocyte Dysfunction

The prevalence of obesity is about tripled between 1975 and 2016 globally (Boutari and Mantzoros 2022), predominantly due to the sedentary lifestyle and unhealthy diet consumption such as refined carbohydrates and high sugar diets. Furthermore, environmental, metabolic, endocrine, and genetic factors are also regarded as the main common causes of obesity in recent decades (Upadhyay et al. 2018; Polyzos and Mantzoros 2019). Specifically, the prevalence of global obesity has increased by nearly 2% points per decade (NCD Risk Factor Collaboration 2017). According to World Health Organization (2023a), they are more than 1 billion people are obese globally including 39 million children, 340 million adolescents, and 650 million adults. Approximately 167 million adults and children are expected to become less healthy due to obesity or overweight by 2025 (World Health Organization 2023a). The prevalence of obesity has increased rapidly between 1980 and 2019 from 3.2 to 12.2% in men. While in women, the prevalence of obesity increased from 6 to 15.7%. The females are continuously demonstrated in terms of the proportions of

B. L. Tan, M. E. Norhaizan, *Nutrients and Oxidative Stress: Biochemistry Aspects and Pharmacological Insights*, SpringerBriefs in Food, Health, and Nutrition, https://doi.org/10.1007/978-3-031-75319-0_4

obesity due to the biologically driven higher percentage of body fat (Wells et al. 2012; Mathew et al. 2018). People with obese or overweight increase their risk developing of nonalcoholic fatty liver disease, cardiovascular disease (CVD), type 2 diabetes, coronary heart disease, stroke, hypertension, inflammatory disturbances, and cancer (Tan et al. 2018a). Elderly people and women were found to have a greater likelihood of obesity (Saha et al. 2023).

Inflammatory cytokines are found in many fat cells; they are linked to all indices of obesity, especially abdominal obesity, and are involved in fat metabolism (Henning 2021). The association between metabolic disturbances and excessive nutrient uptake (lipids, sugars, and fatty acids) is mediated by many types of cells including adipocytes and infiltrating or resident immune cells such as mast cells, monocytes, macrophages, and T cells, which indirectly alter adipocyte dysfunction and function (Kawai et al. 2021). A previous study has shown that dietary fatty acids stimulate protease-activated receptor 2 (PAR2) expression, a biomarker for obesity and a key contributor to inflammation and metabolic dysfunction (Lim et al. 2013).

Another key contributor that enhances a prooxidant environment in obesity is the modulation of proinflammatory response (Tan and Norhaizan 2021a). Inflammation can contribute to oxidative stress in *in vivo* models when there is a marked elevation of free radical generation by immune cells (Zha et al. 2022). Obesity is associated with the alteration of T-cell subsets linked to adipose tissues and the stimulation of infiltration of macrophages into the adipose tissue (Jacks and Lumeng 2024). This phenomenon promotes the production of several proinflammatory cytokines by mature adipocytes, preadipocytes, and immune cells (Palhinha et al. 2019). Increased oxidative stress is associated with chronic inflammation; other sources may also further increase the generation of proinflammatory cytokines in a "vicious cycle". Reactive oxygen species (ROS) enhances the proinflammatory cytokine IL-6 and monocyte chemotactic protein-1 (MCP-1) expression. This process further promotes macrophage infiltration and subsequently results in the proinflammatory environment in the adipose tissue. ROS can also trigger the NF-κB signaling pathway that stimulates TNF-α and IL-6 (Tan et al. 2018a).

In general, adipose tissues are categorized into two classes, namely brown adipose tissue (BAT) and white adipose tissue (WAT) (Dong et al. 2023). Of all types of cells present in WAT, adipocytes are one of the most abundant cells. Several studies found that adipose tissue is characterized by an increased infiltration of macrophages, implied that inflammation may present in adipose tissues (Ni et al. 2020; Jia et al. 2020; Liu et al. 2020). The macrophage infiltration may cause dysregulation in the adipose tissue endocrine system and activate the generation of inflammatory cytokines, thereby leading to endothelial dysfunction and insulin resistance (Kawai et al. 2021). Adipocytes constantly elevate TNF-α expression, in which the adipocytes are significantly increased with obesity (Tan and Norhaizan 2019a; Guerreiro et al. 2022). TNF-α stimulates the cellular kinase complex and thereby activates the NF-κB. Subsequently, this transcription factor modulates the proinflammatory cytokines production such as IL-6 and IL-1β (Vincenzi et al. 2021).

Substantial evidence has suggested that elevated oxidative stress in obesity can decrease the antioxidant defense system and promote superoxide generation by

NADPH oxidase (Zhou et al. 2021). NADPH oxidase is primarily used by neutrophils to generate superoxide to inhibit fungi and invading bacteria. It is activated by advanced glycation end products (AGEs), which are produced after intakes of a high-glucose diet (Cepas et al. 2020). Intriguingly, obesity is inversely linked to glutathione peroxidase 1 (GPx1), superoxide dismutase (SOD), and catalase in the adipose tissues, but not in the skeletal muscle or liver (Savini et al. 2013). However, it remains unknown why the decrease of antioxidant enzymes is only found in adipose tissues. It could be attributed to the high oxidative stress that results in the suppression of the antioxidant enzyme, suggesting that the increase of oxidative stress associated with obesity may cause by an alteration in fat. Collectively, obesity and systemic oxidative stress-related high-fat diet may enhance metabolic dysfunction and inflammation.

Obesity has been shown to promote the development of insulin resistance. Nonetheless, not all obese individuals develop insulin resistance or type 2 diabetes mellitus, imply that the mode of action underlying the association between insulin resistance and obesity must be well-controlled under certain circumstances (Styskal et al. 2012). Indeed, obesity has become an epidemic and represents the predominant risk factor for many chronic diseases such as CVD, cancer, and diabetes (World Health Organization 2016a). Hence, the detrimental impact of oxidative stress on cancer, type 2 diabetes, and CVD outcomes will be described in the following section.

4.2   Type 2 Diabetes

Diabetes is a chronic metabolic disorder affecting nearly 537 million adults (20–79 years) worldwide in 2021 (International Diabetes Federation 2021), with approximately half of all deaths attributable to high blood glucose (World Health Organization 2016b). The total number of people living with diabetes is projected to increase to 643 million by 2030 and 783 million by 2045 (International Diabetes Federation 2021). Type 2 diabetes mellitus is characterized by an inability of the pancreatic β cells to generate enough insulin to maintain glycemic control (Krentz and Gloyn 2020). Diabetes mellitus is a progressive and complex disease that is accompanied by many complications including macro- and microvascular damage, neuropathy, nephropathy, and retinopathy (Paul et al. 2020).

Oxidative stress has been identified as a predominant risk factor in the development of diabetes (Singh et al. 2022). Many risk factors such as unhealthy dietary intake, obesity, and increased age all contribute to an oxidative environment that may alter insulin sensitivity either through the impairment of glucose tolerance or the increase of insulin resistance (Rains and Jain 2011). The modes of action that implicate this disease are complex and involve many cell signaling pathways. Hyperglycemia is associated with diabetes and thereby leads to its progression and an overall oxidative environment (Papachristoforou et al. 2020). Micro- and macrovascular complications lead to the mortality and morbidity of diabetic patients, and all these factors are linked to oxidative stress (Cade 2008).

Insulin resistance plays a crucial role in the progression and development of metabolic dysfunction related to obesity. Insulin resistance occurs when there is an interruption in the insulin signaling cascade caused by the mutation and structural modification in the insulin signaling pathway (Tan and Norhaizan 2021b). The data from animal studies has revealed that homozygous interruption of IRS1 level in mice leads to mild insulin resistance (Yamauchi et al. 1996); whereas the phosphorylation of IRS2 levels in rodents results in severe insulin resistance (Toyoshima et al. 2020).

In terms of insulin resistance and the progression of type 2 diabetes, overnutrition leads to the generation of reactive oxygen species (ROS) and reactive nitrogen species (RNS), thereby increasing oxidative stress in tissues, organs, and cells. Subsequently, oxygen-based free radicals and nitric oxide (NO) damage DNA, proteins, and cell membrane structures, while also modulating transcriptional activity through redox chemistry, including NF-κB, contributing to chronic inflammation and cell apoptosis (Tan et al. 2018a). Elevation of inflammation, increased Ca^{2+} levels, mitochondrial dysfunction, and advanced glycation end products (AGEs) further promote oxidative stress and redox dysregulation in type 2 diabetes (Verdile et al. 2015).

Reduced capacity in the scavenging of free radicals is the primary avenue for ROS generation (Sadiq 2023). GSH is a free radical scavenger that is generated when there is a decrease in glutathione disulphide (GSSG) by glutathione reductase. In addition, NADPH is an important cofactor for glutathione reductase activity (Gansemer et al. 2020). The metabolic pathways used NADPH to modulate the overnutrition or hyperglycemia, and subsequently reducing the cell capacity to produce GSH. For instance, glucose is reduced to sorbitol by aldose reductase during polyol pathway flux. Ultimately, sorbitol is converted by sorbitol dehydrogenase into fructose (El-Kabbani et al. 2004). Although aldose reductase has a low affinity to glucose, their activities are elevated under hyperglycemic circumstances, and subsequently more NADPH is consumed. Decreased GSH levels can cause type 2 diabetes and this phenomenon could be due to the lack of essential amino acids that are required to synthesize GSH or the damage of protein turnover (De Luca et al. 2001). In support of this, the reduction of GSSG levels in Alzheimer's disease patients is associated with the decline of cognitive function. Taken together, inflammation plays a crucial role in type 2 diabetes and insulin resistance. High carbohydrate and saturated fat intake influence insulin secretion. Intracellular signaling pathways in type 2 diabetes, for instance, oxidative stress, active inflammatory process, and aberrant redox modulation may detrimental to insulin secretion and their signaling.

Pancreatic islets with highly specialized and vascularized structures to control the nutrients in the bloodstream and predominantly consist of five cell types, namely ghrelin cells (γ cells), δ cells, β cells, α cells, and pancreatic peptide- (PP-) secreting cells (Wierup et al. 2014). Islets produce blood from the pancreaticoduodenal arteries and splenic branches and interact to elevate dietary nutrients to secrete insulin from β and α cells into the blood circulation and glucagon (during nutrient-deprived conditions including fasting and starvation) (Newsholme et al. 2014). The pancreatic β cell response to glucose depends on the acute modulation of extracellular or intracellular RNS and ROS (Newsholme et al. 2012; Gray and Heart 2010). Increased glycolytic flux boosts ATP generation and oxidative phosphorylation, and thereby leads to the formation of $O_2^{\cdot-}$ released from the electron transport chain (Schoonbroodt and Piette 2000). High glucose levels may promote ROS via several possible modes of action, for instance, the production of glucose autoxidation and advanced glycation end products (AGEs) (Verdile et al. 2015).

Alteration of the structure via hyperphosphorylation of serine at residues Ser[307], Ser[632], Ser[602], and Ser[612] in IRS1 has been suggested to be an important mechanistic element that is responsible for the increase of insulin resistance in rodents (Saini 2010). Elevated protein expression, for instance, TNF-α and c-Jun N-terminal kinase 1 (JNK1), could be derived from the adipose expansion and can induce serine hyperphosphorylation of IRS1, particularly at residue Ser[636]. Nevertheless, it remains unknown whether the individual residues or combination of residues need to be hyperphosphorylated to improve insulin-resistant phenotype.

Compelling evidence has suggested an association between increased carbonylation and nitrosylation of protein in insulin- or obese-resistant phenotypes and insulin-sensitive tissues (Ovadia et al. 2011; Muellenbach et al. 2009; Muellenbach et al. 2008), suggesting that an insulin-resistant phenotype may boost the decrease of insulin receptor level. Collectively, the progression and development of diabetes mellitus are linked to β cell dysfunction and insulin resistance, and this process is often linked to obesity (Newsholme et al. 2014).

4.3 Cardiovascular Disease

Cardiovascular disease (CVD) has become the leading cause of death worldwide, contributing to about 17.9 million lives each year (World Health Organization 2023b). CVD is a cluster of heart and blood vessel disorders, such as rheumatic heart disease, coronary heart disease, and cerebrovascular disease (World Health Organization 2023b). One third of CVD deaths have occurred prematurely in people below 70 years old, and more than four out of five CVD deaths are due to strokes and heart attacks (World Health Organization 2023b).

Oxidative stress plays an important role in the development and progression of CVD. CVD is attributed to lifestyle factors, especially sedentary lifestyles, smoking, dietary intake, and alcohol consumption. Western dietary habits that are low in dietary fiber and high in fat increase the incidence of CVD. Low-grade and chronic inflammation has been shown as a major pathophysiology in obesity and other related diseases including CVD (Tan et al. 2018a). C-reactive protein (CRP) has been demonstrated as an independent risk factor for the development of CVD (Koziarska-Rościszewska et al. 2021). Increased CRP in obesity could be due to the macrophage infiltration into expanded adipose tissue and thereby results in the generation and release of macrophage-derived proinflammatory cytokines, for instance, TNF-α and IL-6 (Scarano et al. 2021).

The initial step of atherosclerosis has been implicated by the attraction or adherence of monocytes to the vascular endothelium and their migration into the vessel wall (Kang et al. 2021). The adhesion molecules, for instance, ICAM-1, selectins, and VCAM-1 enhance the adhesion of leukocytes to the vascular endothelium (Singh et al. 2023), which in turn induced by inflammatory factors such as TNF-α, interleukin-1 (IL-1), and CRP (Benincasa et al. 2022). VCAM-1 interacts with specific leukocytes in nascent atheroma. Both macrophages and endothelial cells produce ICAM-1 in response to inflammatory cytokines, for instance, TNF-α, interferon-γ, and IL-1 (Wiesolek et al. 2020).

The development of lesions is characterized by the migration of smooth muscle cells from the medial layer of the artery wall into subendothelial space (Milutinović et al. 2020). Smooth muscle cells migrate and proliferate with the facilitation of some growth factors and cytokines generated by inflammatory and endothelial cells (Parnigoni et al. 2022). Nevertheless, the smooth muscle cell is a source of inflammatory mediators such as monocyte chemoattractant protein-1 (MCP-1). Mice with a deficiency of MCP-1 expression or its chemokine receptor, CCR2, develop fewer atherosclerotic lesions. Likewise, the initiators of the atherosclerotic cascade, for instance, ox-LDL, were demonstrated to enhance the growth factors production such as macrophage colony-stimulating factor (M-CSF) (Wu et al. 2017).

The activation of inflammatory cells and smooth muscle cells is associated with the release of mediators, for instance, cytokines, growth factors, and adhesion molecules (Beck-Joseph and Lehoux 2021). IL-6 increases the plasminogen activator inhibitor type 1, plasma CRP levels, and fibrinogen, which in turn amplify and enhance both inflammatory and procoagulant responses (Foley and Conway 2016).

One common characteristic of CVD is an elevation of oxidative stress in the heart (Donia and Khamis 2021). In particular, systemic oxidative damage in patients with CVD was attributed to decrease antioxidant defense and ROS accumulation (Dubois-Deruy et al. 2020). Ilkun and Boudina (2013) show that an high-fat diet (HFD) promotes ROS production and decreased antioxidant capacity, thereby leading to many disorders such as endothelial dysfunction, which is characterized by a reduced bioavailability of vasodilators, namely nitric oxide (NO), and increased endothelium-derived contractile factors leading to atherosclerotic disease. The mechanisms underlying cardiac pathology are complex and include increased oxidative stress, abnormal autophagy, modified calcium homeostasis, mitochondrial dysfunction, increased stiffness and fibrosis, and lipid accumulation. Taken together, extramitochondrial and mitochondrial sources of ROS and a decrease in antioxidant defense mechanisms have occurred in the animals and human myocardium (Ilkun and Boudina 2013).

4.4 Cancer

Cancer has become the second leading cause of death worldwide, representing approximately 9.6 million deaths in 2018 (World Health Organization 2023c). About 30–50% of cancer deaths could be prevented by implementing existing evidence-based prevention approaches and avoiding or modifying key risk factors. Cancer is a cluster of diseases that can start in almost any tissue or organ of the body when abnormal cells grow uncontrollably. It arises into tumor cells from the transformation of normal cells in a series of processes that usually progress from a precancerous lesion to a malignant tumor (World Health Organization 2023d).

Substantial studies have shown that high oxidative stress results in cancer including colorectal cancer (Tan et al. 2014; Tan and Norhaizan 2019a, b). Oxidative stress is hypothesized to be linked to cancer and obesity. In support of this, an animal-obese model of nonalcoholic steatohepatitis shows that the absence of adiponectin increases oxidative stress and boosts hepatic tumor formation (VanSaun 2013). ROS plays a vital role in the development of cancer (Tan and Norhaizan 2021b). The increased ROS promotes the susceptibility to mutagenic agents or mutation rates and thereby leading to DNA damage during the early phases of carcinogenesis (Costa de Almeida et al. 2021).

The incidence of cancer increases steeply with age. A previous study has shown that a single-cell lineage has occurred before the malignant cells are formed (Quinn et al. 2021). Nevertheless, aging has been suggested as a time-dependent event, and probably the summation of innumerable different processes. Therefore, the time-dependent emergence of cancer may be associated with other age-related conditions (Le et al. 2019). ROS is a hallmark of several types of cancer. Inflammatory cells generate many ROS (Aminjan et al. 2019). The oxygen biochemistry is mediated through the activation of macrophages, neutrophils, and plasma membrane NADPH oxidase, and thereby releases the H_2O_2, hydroxyl radicals, and superoxide anion. Moreover, inflammation interacts via the production of ROS and RNS, and thereby causes oxidative damage in the cellular components (Tan et al. 2018a). Several pro-inflammatory mediators including chemokines, prostaglandins, and cytokines turn on the angiogenesis switches mainly mediated by vascular endothelial growth factors (VEGF) (Fu et al. 2020). Inflammation is an important component of tumor progression (Chakraborty et al. 2020). Indeed, some cancers may arise from sites of chronic irritation, inflammation, and infection (Eyvazi et al. 2020). Data from the previous study revealed that the tumor microenvironment is mainly orchestrated by inflammatory cells, and is an indispensable player in enhancing survival, migration, neoplastic, and proliferation (Neophytou et al. 2021).

Pathological angiogenesis is a hallmark of ischemic, inflammatory diseases, and cancer (La Mendola et al. 2022). Inflammation in the tumor microenvironment is characterized by leukocyte infiltration, ranging from distribution, composition, and size, such as mast cells, natural killer (NK) cells, eosinophils, tumor-associated macrophages (TAM), dendritic cells, neutrophils, and lymphocytes (Tiwari et al. 2022). These cells produce several cytotoxic mediators such as ROS and RNS, serine proteases and cysteine, matrix metalloproteinase (MMP), interferons (IFNs), interleukins (IL-6, IL-8, and IL-1), and enzymes including lipooxygenase-5 (LOX-5), phospholipase A2 (PLA2), and cyclooxygenase-2 (COX-2) (Andreou et al. 2020; Tan et al. 2018a, b). Stimulation of activator protein-1 (AP-1) increases cell proliferation by suppressing p21waf protein expression and promoting growth stimulatory transcriptional activity of cyclin D1. It has been shown that AP-1 and

NF-κB, inducible by tumor promoters of oxidative stimuli, demonstrate stimulation in response to differential protein levels or tumor promoters in JB6 cells (Hsu et al. 2000). Many growth factors including insulin-like growth factor I or fibroblast growth factor 2 generate ROS in PANC-1 and MIA PaCa-2 cells, which are human pancreatic adenocarcinoma cells that increase cell growth (Vaquero et al. 2004). In addition, the oxidative pentose pathway (OPP) and GSH antioxidant defense system play a vital role in the regulation of gastrointestinal and colon cancer apoptosis and cell proliferation (Matthews et al. 2006). The OPP provides NADPH for the mediation of intracellular redox status and synthesis of GSH, which is responsible for the inactivation of intracellular ROS and subsequently triggers apoptosis and leads to cell injury. Depletion of GSH promotes the sensitivity of cells against ROS. Hence, inhibition of the OPP and/or GSH defense system may enhance the sensitivity of gastric and colon cancer cells to anticancer therapy. The enzymatic product of thymidine phosphorylase (TP) generates ROS within cancer cells that modulate the growth of colon cancer cells (Paladhi et al. 2022).

An earlier study has shown that insulin is a proliferation factor for prostate cancer; hence, the decreased of carbohydrates may thereby reduce serum insulin and decrease the growth of prostate cancer (Lubik and Gunter 2011). Intriguingly, data from epidemiological studies found that patients with obesity and type 2 diabetes show a greater likelihood of breast, liver, pancreatic, and colorectal cancers (Yang and Chan 2012; Shi and Hu 2014). These data suggest that adiponectin, leptin, inflammation, and insulin/insulin-like growth factor-1 are additive between obesity or type 2 diabetes and cancers. Accumulation of fat is usually associated with systemic oxidative stress through increased of ROS (Tan et al. 2018a). Increased oxidative stress can result in chronic inflammation, and thereby could mediate chronic disease including cancer (Tan et al. 2018a). Oxidative stress can induce many transcriptional factors including NF-κB, Wnt/β-catenin, and nuclear factor E2-related factor 2 (*Nrf2*) and thus stimulates inflammatory pathways (Tan et al. 2018a). Collectively, the evidence suggests that elevated local or circulating ROS levels derived from the expansion of the adipose tissue in a tumor environment promote oxidative stress within cancer cells and subsequently result in an increased risk for the progression of cancer in patients with obesity or type 2 diabetes.

References

Aminjan HH, Abtahi SR, Hazrati E et al (2019) Targeting of oxidative stress and inflammation through ROS/NF-kappaB pathway in phosphine-induced hepatotoxicity mitigation. Life Sci 232:116607

Andreou N-P, Legaki E, Gazouli M (2020) Inflammatory bowel disease pathobiology: the role of the interferon signature. Ann Gastroenterol 33:125–133

Beck-Joseph J, Lehoux S (2021) Molecular interactions between vascular smooth muscle cells and macrophages in atherosclerosis. Front Cardiovasc Med 8(8):737934

Benincasa G, Coscioni E, Napoli C (2022) Cardiovascular risk factors and molecular routes underlying endothelial dysfunction: novel opportunities for primary prevention. Biochem Pharmacol 202:115108

Boutari C, Mantzoros CS (2022) A 2022 update on the epidemiology of obesity and a call to action: as its twin COVID-19 pandemic appears to be receding, the obesity and dysmetabolism pandemic continues to rage on. Metabolism 133:155217

Cade WT (2008) Diabetes-related microvascular and macrovascular diseases in the physical therapy setting. Phys Ther 88:1322–1335

Cepas V, Collino M, Mayo JC et al (2020) Redox signaling and advanced glycation endproducts (AGEs) in diet-related diseases. Antioxidants 9:142

Chakraborty C, Sharma AR, Sharma G et al (2020) The interplay among miRNAs, major cytokines, and cancer-related inflammation. Mol Ther Nucleic Acids 20:606–620

Costa de Almeida L, Calil FA, Machado-Neto JA et al (2021) DNA damaging agents and DNA repair: from carcinogenesis to cancer therapy. Cancer Genet 252–253:6–24

De Luca G, Calpona PR, Caponetti A et al (2001) Preliminary report: amino acid profile in platelets of diabetic patients. Metabolism 50:739–741

Dong H, Qin M, Wang P et al (2023) Regulatory effects and mechanisms of exercise on activation of brown adipose tissue (BAT) and browning of white adipose tissue (WAT). Adipocytes 12:2266147

Donia T, Khamis A (2021) Management of oxidative stress and inflammation in cardiovascular diseases: mechanisms and challenges. Environ Sci Pollut Res 28:34121–34153

Dubois-Deruy E, Peugnet V, Turkieh A et al (2020) Oxidative stress in cardiovascular diseases. Antioxidants 9:864

El-Kabbani O, Darmanin C, Chung RP-T (2004) Sorbitol dehydrogenase: structure, function and ligand design. Curr Med Chem 11:465–476

Eyvazi S, Vostakolaei MA, Dilmaghani A et al (2020) The oncogenic roles of bacterial infections in development of cancer. Microb Pathog 141:104019

Foley JH, Conway EM (2016) Cross talk pathways between coagulation and inflammation. Circ Res 118:1392–1408

Fu L-Q, Du W-L, Cai M-H et al (2020) The roles of tumor-associated macrophages in tumor angiogenesis and metastasis. Cell Immunol 353:104119

Gansemer ER, McCommis KS, Martino M et al (2020) NADPH and glutathione redox link TCA cycle activity to endoplasmic reticulum homeostasis. iScience 23:101116

Gray JP, Heart E (2010) Usurping the mitochondrial supremacy: extra mitochondrial sources of reactive oxygen intermediates and their role in beta cell metabolism and insulin secretion. Toxicol Mech Methods 20:167–174

Guerreiro VA, Carvalho D, Freitas P (2022) Obesity, adipose tissue, and inflammation answered in questions. J Obes 2022., Article ID 2252516:11

Henning RJ (2021) Obesity and obesity-induced inflammatory disease contribute to atherosclerosis: a review of the pathophysiology and treatment of obesity. Am J Cardiovasc Dis 11:504–529

Hsu TC, Young MR, Cmarik J et al (2000) Activator protein 1 (AP-1)- and nuclear factor kappaB (NF-kappaB)-dependent transcriptional events in carcinogenesis. Free Radic Biol Med 28:1338–1348

Ilkun O, Boudina S (2013) Cardiac dysfunction and oxidative stress in the metabolic syndrome: an update on antioxidant therapies. Curr Pharm Design 19:4806–4817

International Diabetes Federation (2021) Diabetes facts and figures. https://idf.org/aboutdiabetes/what-is-diabetes/facts-figures.html. Accessed 19 Feb 2023

Jacks RD, Lumeng CN (2024) Macrophage and T cell networks in adipose tissue. Nat Rev Endocrinol 20:50–61

Jia Q, Morgan-Bathke ME, Jensen MD (2020) Adipose tissue macrophage burden, systemic inflammation, and insulin resistance. Am J Physiol Endocrinol Metab 319:E254–E264

Kang H, Li X, Xiong K et al (2021) The entry and egress of monocytes in atherosclerosis: a biochemical and biomechanical driven process. Cardiovasc Ther 2021., Article ID 6642927:17

Kawai T, Autieri MV, Scalia R (2021) Adipose tissue inflammation and metabolic dysfunction in obesity. Am J Physiol Cell Physiol 320:C375–C391

Koziarska-Rościszewska M, Gluba-Brzózka A, Franczyk B et al (2021) High-sensitivity C-reactive protein relationship with metabolic disorders and cardiovascular diseases risk factors. Life 11:742

Krentz NAJ, Gloyn AL (2020) Insights into pancreatic islet cell dysfunction from type 2 diabetes mellitus genetics. Nat Rev Endocrinol 16:202–212

La Mendola D, Trincavelli ML, Martini C (2022) Angiogenesis in disease. Int J Mol Sci 23:10962

Le A, Udupa S, Zhang C (2019) The metabolic interplay between cancer and other diseases. Trends Cancer 5:809–821

Lim J, Iyer A, Liu L et al (2013) Diet-induced obesity, adipose inflammation, and metabolic dysfunction correlating with PAR2 expression are attenuated by PAR2 antagonism. FASEB J 27:4757–4767

Liu Y, Lu X, Li X et al (2020) High-fat diet triggers obesity-related early infiltration of macrophages into adipose tissue and transient reduction of blood monocyte count. Mol Immunol 117:139–146

Lubik AA, Gunter JH, Hendy SC et al (2011) Insulin increases *de novo* steroidogenesis in prostate cancer cells. Cancer Res 71:5754–5764

Mathew H, Castracane VD, Mantzoros C (2018) Adipose tissue and reproductive health. Metabolism 86:18–32

Matthews GM, Howarth GS, Butler RN (2006) Nutrient and antioxidant modulation of apoptosis in gastric and colon cancer cells. Cancer Biol Ther 5:569–572

Milutinović A, Šuput D, Zorc-Pleskovič R (2020) Pathogenesis of atherosclerosis in the tunica intima, media, and adventitia of coronary arteries: an updated review. Bosn J Basic Med Sci 20:21–30

Muellenbach EA, Diehl CJ, Teachey MK et al (2008) Interactions of the advanced glycation end product inhibitor pyridoxamine and the antioxidant alpha-lipoic acid on insulin resistance in the obese Zucker rat. Metabolism 57:1465–1472

Muellenbach EM, Diehl CJ, Teachey MK et al (2009) Metabolic interactions of AGE inhibitor pyridoxamine and antioxidant α-lipoic acid following 22 weeks of treatment in obese Zucker rats. Life Sci 84:563–568

NCD Risk Factor Collaboration (NCD-RisC) (2017) Worldwide trends in body-mass index, underweight, overweight, and obesity from 1975 to 2016: a pooled analysis of 2416 population-based measurement studies in 128·9 million children, adolescents, and adults. Lancet (London, England) 390:2627–2642

Neophytou CM, Panagi M, Stylianopoulos T et al (2021) The role of tumor microenvironment in cancer metastasis: molecular mechanisms and therapeutic opportunities. Cancers 13:2053

Newsholme P, Rebelato E, Abdulkader F et al (2012) Reactive oxygen and nitrogen species generation, antioxidant defenses, and β-cell function: a critical role for amino acids. J Endocrinol 214:11–20

Newsholme P, Cruzat V, Arfuso F et al (2014) Nutrient regulation of insulin secretion and action. J Endocrinol 221:R105–R120

Ni Y, Ni L, Zhuge F et al (2020) Adipose tissue macrophage phenotypes and characteristics: the key to insulin resistance in obesity and metabolic disorders. Obesity 28:225–234

Ovadia H, Haim Y, Nov O et al (2011) Increased adipocyte-Snitrosylation targets anti-lipolytic action of insulin relevance to adipose tissue dysfunction in obesity. J Biol Chem 286:30433–30443

Paladhi A, Daripa S, Mondal I et al (2022) Targeting thymidine phosphorylase alleviates resistance to dendritic cell immunotherapy in colorectal cancer and promotes antitumor immunity. Front Immunol 13:988071

Palhinha L, Liechocki S, Hottz ED et al (2019) Leptin induces proadipogenic and proinflammatory signaling in adipocytes. Front Endocrinol 10:841

Papachristoforou E, Lambadiari V, Maratou E et al (2020) Association of glycemic indices (hyperglycemia, glucose variability, and hypoglycemia) with oxidative stress and diabetic complications. J Diabetes Res. Article ID 7489795

Parnigoni A, Viola M, Karousou E et al (2022) Hyaluronan in pathophysiology of vascular diseases: specific roles in smooth muscle cells, endothelial cells, and macrophages. Am J Physiol Cell Physiol 323:C505–C519

Paul S, Ali A, Katare R (2020) Molecular complexities underlying the vascular complications of diabetes mellitus–a comprehensive review. J Diabetes Complicat 34:107613

Polyzos SA, Mantzoros CS (2019) Obesity: seize the day, fight the fat. Metabolism 92:1–5

Quinn JJ, Jones MG, Okimoto RA et al (2021) Single-cell lineages reveal the rates, routes, and drivers of metastasis in cancer xenografts. Science 371:eabc1944

Rains JL, Jain SK (2011) Oxidative stress, insulin signaling and diabetes. Free Radic Biol Med 50:567–575

Sadiq IZ (2023) Free radicals and oxidative stress: signaling mechanisms, redox basis for human diseases, and cell cycle regulation. Curr Mol Med 23:13–35

Saha A, Mandal B, Muhammad T et al (2023) Gender-specific determinants of overweight and obesity among older adults in India: evidence from a cross-sectional survey, 2017–18. BMC Public Health 23:2313

Saini V (2010) Molecular mechanisms of insulin resistance in type 2 diabetes mellitus. World J Diabetes 1:68–75

Savini I, Catani MV, Evangelista D et al (2013) Obesity-associated oxidative stress: strategies finalized to improve redox state. Int J Mol Sci 14:10497–10538

Scarano F, Gliozzi M, Zito MC et al (2021) Potential of nutraceutical supplementation in the modulation of white and brown fat tissues in obesity-associated disorders: role of inflammatory signalling. Int J Mol Sci 22:3351

Schoonbroodt S, Piette J (2000) Oxidative stress interference with the nuclear factor-κB activation pathways. Biochem Pharmacol 60:1075–1083

Shi Y, Hu FB (2014) The global implications of diabetes and cancer. Lancet 383:1947–1948

Singh A, Kukreti R, Saso L et al (2022) Mechanistic insight into oxidative stress-triggered signaling pathways and type 2 diabetes. Molecules 27:950

Singh V, Kaur R, Kumari P et al (2023) ICAM-1 and VCAM-1: gatekeepers in various inflammatory and cardiovascular disorders. Clin Chim Acta 548:117487

Styskal J, Remmen HV, Richardson A et al (2012) Oxidative stress and diabetes: what can we learn about insulin resistance from antioxidant mutant mouse models? Free Radic Biol Med 52:46–58

Su X, Peng D (2020) Adipokines as novel biomarkers of cardio-metabolic disorders. Clin Chim Acta 507:31–38

Tan BL, Norhaizan ME (2019a) Effect of high-fat diets on oxidative stress, cellular inflammatory response and cognitive function. Nutrients 11:2579

Tan BL, Norhaizan ME (2019b) *Manilkara zapota* (L.) P. Royen leaf water extract triggered apoptosis and activated caspase-dependent pathway in HT-29 human colorectal cancer cell line. Biomed Pharmacol 110:748–757

Tan BL, Norhaizan ME (2021a) Chapter 5 Implications of inflammation in aging and age-related diseases. In: Tan BL, Norhaizan ME (eds) The role of antioxidants in longevity and age-related diseases. Springer Nature, Cham, pp 51–80

Tan BL, Norhaizan ME (2021b) Chapter 3 Age-related oxidative stress-induced redox imbalance. In: Tan BL, Norhaizan ME (eds) The role of antioxidants in longevity and age-related diseases. Springer Nature, Cham, pp 27–38

Tan BL, Norhaizan ME, Rahman HS et al (2014) Brewers' rice induces apoptosis in azoxymethane-induced colon carcinogenesis in rats via suppression of cell proliferation and the Wnt signaling pathway. BMC Complement Altern Med 14:304

Tan BL, Norhaizan ME, Liew W-P-P (2018a) Nutrients and oxidative stress: friend or foe? Oxid Med Cell Longev 2018., Article ID 9719584:24

Tan BL, Norhaizan ME, Liew W-P-P et al (2018b) Antioxidant and oxidative stress: a mutual interplay in age-related diseases. Front Pharmacol 9:1162

Tiwari A, Trivedi R, Lin S-Y (2022) Tumor microenvironment: barrier or opportunity towards effective cancer therapy. J Biomed Sci 29:83

Toyoshima Y, Nakamura K, Tokita R et al (2020) Disruption of insulin receptor substrate-2 impairs growth but not insulin function in rats. J Biol Chem 295:11914–11927

Upadhyay J, Farr O, Perakakis N et al (2018) Obesity as a disease. Med Clin North Am 102:13–33

VanSaun MN (2013) Molecular pathways: adiponentin and leptin signaling in cancer. Clin Cancer Res 19:1926–1932

Vaquero EC, Edderkaoui M, Pandol SJ et al (2004) Reactive oxygen species produced by NAD(P) H oxidase inhibit apoptosis in pancreatic cancer cells. J Biol Chem 279:34643–34654

Verdile G, Keane KN, Cruzat VF et al (2015) Inflammation and oxidative stress: the molecular connectivity between insulin resistance, obesity, and Alzheimer's disease. Mediators Inflamm., Article ID 105828:17

Vincenzi A, Goettert MI, de Souza CFV (2021) An evaluation of the effects of probiotics on tumoral necrosis factor (TNF-α) signaling and gene expression. Cytokine Growth Factor Rev 57:27–38

Wells JCK, Marphatia AA, Cole TJ et al (2012) Associations of economic and gender inequality with global obesity prevalence: understanding the female excess. Soc Sci Med 75:482–490

Wierup N, Sundler F, Heller RS (2014) The islet ghrelin cell. J Mol Endocrinol 52:R35–R49

Wiesolek HL, Bui TM, Lee JJ et al (2020) Intercellular adhesion molecule 1 functions as an efferocytosis receptor in inflammatory macrophages. Am J Pathol 190:P874–P885

World Health Organization (2016a) Obesity http://www.who.int/topics/obesity/en/

World Health Organization (2016b) Global report on diabetes. World Health Organization, Geneva

World Health Organization (2023a) World Obesity Day 2022–Accelerating action to stop obesity. https://www.who.int/news/item/04-03-2022-world-obesity-day-2022-accelerating-action-to-stop-obesity. Accessed 9 Feb 2023

World Health Organization (2023b) Cardiovascular diseases. https://wwwwhoint/health-topics/cardiovascular-diseases#tab=tab_1 Accessed 20 Feb 2023

World Health Organization (2023c) Cancer. https://www.who.int/health-topics/cancer#tab=tab_1. Accessed 21 Feb 2023

World Health Organization (2023d) World Cancer Day 2023. https://www.emro.who.int/noncommunicable-diseases/campaigns/world-cancer-day-2023.html. Accessed 21 Feb 2023

Wu M-Y, Li C-J, Hou M-F et al (2017) New insights into the role of inflammation in the pathogenesis of atherosclerosis. Int J Mol Sci 18:2034

Yamauchi T, Tobe K, Tamemoto H et al (1996) Insulin signalling and insulin actions in the muscles and livers of insulin-resistant, insulin receptor substrate 1-deficient mice. Mol Cell Biol 16:3074–3084

Yang X-L, Chan JCN (2012) Diabetes, insulin and cancer risk. World J Diabetes 3:60–64

Zha Z, Liu S, Liu Y et al (2022) Potential utility of natural products against oxidative stress in animal models of multiple sclerosis. Antioxidants 11:1495

Zhao Q, Zhu L, Wang S et al (2023) Molecular mechanism of the anti-inflammatory effects of plant essential oils: a systematic review. J Ethnopharmacol 301:115829

Zhou Y, Li H, Xia N (2021) The interplay between adipose tissue and vasculature: role of oxidative stress in obesity. Front Cardiovasc Med 8:650214

Chapter 5
High Carbohydrates Intake and Type 2 Diabetes

5.1 Diabetes Mellitus

Diabetes mellitus is defined by postprandial hyperglycemia (plasma glucose more than 11.1 mM 2 h after an oral glucose tolerance test) or the presence of fasting hyperglycemia (plasma glucose more than 7.0 mM) (Sakai et al. 2003). Type 2 diabetes is the most prevalent form of disease that often arises in the context of a sedentary lifestyle and obesity with insulin resistance in the adipose tissue, skeletal muscles, and liver. Nonetheless, the disease is developed when the endocrine pancreas fails to fully compensate for insulin resistance. Therefore, despite the varying contributions of insulin secretion deficiency and insulin resistance to hyperglycemia among different patients (Wehinger et al. 2015), a defect in insulin secretion by the endocrine pancreas is necessary for the development of type 2 diabetes (Godoy et al. 2011; Mehmeti et al. 2011; Wu et al. 2017). This defect, caused by alterations in β-cell function and mass, is typically linked to oxidative stress.

5.2 The Role of Endocrine Pancreas in Blood Glucose Homeostasis

The endocrine pancreas, consisting of numerous pancreatic islets of Langerhans dispersed throughout the exocrine pancreas, plays a crucial role in blood glucose homeostasis. The islets are small heterogeneous micro-organs comprised of endocrine cells with a dense capillary network lined by fenestrated endothelial cells (Prentki et al. 2013) and secrete ghrelin (ε-cells), pancreatic polypeptide (γ-cells), somatostatin (δ-cells), glucagon (α-cells), or insulin (β-cells) (Chen et al. 2017). Among all the islet cells, β-cells are the most extensively studied due to their highly

© The Author(s), under exclusive license to Springer Nature Switzerland AG 2024   43
B. L. Tan, M. E. Norhaizan, *Nutrients and Oxidative Stress: Biochemistry Aspects and Pharmacological Insights*, SpringerBriefs in Food, Health, and Nutrition, https://doi.org/10.1007/978-3-031-75319-0_5

relative accessibility and abundance, their vital role in the development of type 2 and type 1 diabetes (Roma and Jonas 2020), and the importance of insulin in decreasing the blood glucose levels rapidly while favoring anabolic pathways after meals.

Pancreatic β-cells are highly specialized cells that constantly adapt the insulin secretion rate to the plasma concentration of glucose and other nutrients, due to the unique coupling system between changes in insulin granule exocytosis, insulin biosynthesis, and nutrient metabolism (Scharfmann et al. 2013). This coupling system involves the acceleration of mitochondrial metabolism and glycolysis with rapid changes in the oxidation state of some redox couples such as an increase in NADPH/NADP$^+$ and NADH/NAD$^+$ ratios, and is likely to be linked to the increased generation of $\cdot O_2^-$. Emerging evidence revealed that mitochondria play a crucial role in β-cells production of metabolic coupling factors such as H_2O_2 (Tan and Norhaizan 2021).

5.3 High Carbohydrates Intakes and Oxidative Stress

Empirical evidence reveals that high consumption of macronutrients can increase oxidative stress and thereby contribute to inflammation through nuclear factor-kappa B (NF-κB) signaling pathways. Dietary carbohydrate consumption has drawn interest among researchers due to the relationship between a high glycemic load (GL) or glycemic index (GI) diet with cancer, diabetes, coronary heart disease, and obesity. High GL diets have been characterized as a common characteristic of Western culture; they are heavy in refined carbohydrates and added sugars. On the other hand, low GI foods were demonstrated to reduce postprandial glycemia in type 2 diabetes and obese/overweight patients (Zafar et al. 2019). Consistent associations between diabetes and high GI have been reported in both cohort and observational studies (Lal et al. 2021).

The high GI of white rice may contribute to high oxidative stress. Indeed, Asian populations consume large amounts of rice as a staple food. Therefore, dietary carbohydrate consumption plays an important role in the development of metabolic diseases in Asian populations. Likewise, data from a population-based study also reported a positive relationship between diabetes and total carbohydrates and rice intake in Japanese women (Nanri et al. 2010; Hu et al. 2012). In addition to the effects observed in diabetes, high consumption of refined grain was also found to be positively associated with triglycerides and fasting blood glucose levels and negatively linked to high-density lipoprotein (HDL) cholesterol in Korean and Indian populations (Radhika et al. 2009; Song et al. 2014), implied that a high GI diet may negatively impact health.

The prevalence of metabolic syndrome has increased considerably due to the excessive intake of carbohydrates including fructose and/or sucrose. An animal study has demonstrated that chronic consumption of sucrose and fructose exacerbates metabolic syndrome-induced cardiac hypertrophy which is linked to higher oxidative stress and calcium/calmodulin-dependent protein kinase type II subunit delta oxidation (ox-CaMKIIδ) and oxidative stress (Arias-Chávez et al. 2022). The study by Adedeji et al. (2022) further demonstrated that feeding rats with a high carbohydrate diet increased malondialdehyde (MDA) concentrations.

Excessive consumption of calories from either a high-fat or high-carbohydrate diet can lead to more substrates to access mitochondrial respiration (Teodoro et al. 2013). Ultimately, the number of electrons donated to the electron transport chain may elevate (Brownlee 2001). The extra electron may back up at complex III when reaching a threshold voltage, which further donations to molecular oxygen, and generates high superoxide levels (Brownlee 2001).

Notably, excessive high intakes of carbohydrates may result in the downregulation of insulin receptor transcriptional factors and decreased insulin binding in the skeletal muscle (Catena et al. 2003). High levels of glucose and insulin may reduce the insulin binding to insulin receptors in adipocytes (Burén et al. 2003), which negatively mediates Akt activity. The decreased antioxidant capacity or accumulation of RNS/ROS due to the elevation of carbohydrate metabolism in insulin target tissues may alter the phosphorylation status of the signaling pathways, therefore leading to deactivation. Furthermore, exposure to hydrogen peroxide (H_2O_2) reduces glucose transport in adipocytes and muscles *in vitro* and stimulates a significant loss in proximal and distal insulin signaling (Henriksen et al. 2011).

Emerging studies from epidemiological showed that intakes of refined carbohydrates, for instance, fructose-rich syrups, potentially result in obesity and epidemics of type 2 diabetes (DiNicolantonio et al. 2015; Hu and Malik 2010). Fructose-rich syrups may also potentially lead to CVD and diabetes risk (DiNicolantonio et al. 2015). The animal study found that the administration of normal rats with fructose-rich diets may trigger metabolic and endocrine derangements, interfering with several tissues and organs (Alzamendi et al. 2009; Francini et al. 2010). As the liver is vital for fructose uptake and metabolism, few studies are centered on the metabolism of hepatic glucose (Castro et al. 2014). Despite the molecular mechanism associated with the metabolism of carbohydrates and the detrimental effects of fructose, several studies demonstrated that oxidative stress could play a critical role (Castro et al. 2012, 2015). Administration of fructose is likely to cause inflammation *in vivo* (Alzamendi et al. 2009). This study shows the relationship between fructose and insulin resistance and its role in carbohydrate metabolism and hepatic metabolism against anabolic pathway and impaired glucose tolerance (Francini et al. 2010; Castro et al. 2011, 2012). Furthermore, fructose may mediate the liver glucokinase activity through ROS generation (Castro et al. 2014). These findings imply that several metabolic alterations triggered by fructose in the liver are more likely to be initiated by fructokinase to elevate the phosphorylation of fructose, and thus via adaptive changes that attempt to convert the substrate flow to energy storage from mitochondrial metabolism (Castro et al. 2014).

5.4 Carbohydrate Intake and Type 2 Diabetes

Epidemiological studies have demonstrated the causal relationship between metabolic diseases and fructose consumption including type 2 diabetes. A prospective cohort study demonstrated that individuals who consumed more than one sweetened beverage daily showed an 83% higher risk of type 2 diabetes compared to individuals drinking less than one beverage daily (Schulze et al. 2004). It has been hypothesized that dietary sugar consumption plays a primary role in the development of type 2 diabetes (Malik et al. 2010; de Koning et al. 2012; Goran et al. 2013; O'Connor et al. 2015), yet the findings are inconsistent (White 2013). The fructose component of high-sugar foods has been demonstrated as a predominant promotor of adverse cardiometabolic health outcomes when excessive consumption (Stanhope et al. 2011; Wang et al. 2014). Compared to dietary glucose, dietary fructose shows a relatively low insulin secretion (Teff et al. 2004, 2009). Previous studies have shown that fructose consumption/substitution can beneficially regulate blood glucose levels (Livesey and Taylor 2008; Evans et al. 2017). Research evidence indicates that fructose-induced fat accumulation leads to insulin resistance and hepatic lipotoxicity (Utzschneider and Kahn 2006). Subsequently, hepatic insulin resistance contributes to hyperlipidemia, lipotoxicity, and lipid accumulation in other organs such as skeletal muscle (Thirunavukkarasu et al. 2004).

The prevalence of type 2 diabetes is 20% higher in countries with higher high-fructose corn syrup availability compared to the low availability of high-fructose corn syrup, independently of the prevalence of obesity (Goran et al. 2013). High-fructose corn syrup, containing about 15% fructose, is developed via enzyme reaction when fructose is converted from glucose by glucose isomerase (Takasaki 1966). Following this, the manufacturers increased the amount of fructose in high-fructose corn syrup. In the 1980s, the fructose content in high-fructose corn syrup was 55%, which is a similar ratio of fructose and glucose to that in sucrose (Hanover and White 1993).

High-fructose corn syrup is commonly used as a predominant sweetener, for instance, in candy, desserts, pastries, and sugar-sweetened beverages, and has been associated with various chronic diseases including diabetes (Hattori et al. 2021). Hattori et al. (2021) assessed excessive consumption of high-fructose corn syrup water on glucose tolerance in male Institute of Cancer Research (ICR) mice. Intriguingly, the data showed that excess high-fructose corn syrup-water intake did not cause obesity, but led to impaired glucose tolerance. The study found that high-fructose corn syrup affects fructose and glucose metabolism, for instance, reduced glucose transporter 2, ketohexokinase, and glucokinases in the pancreas, suggesting that excessive intakes of high-fructose corn syrup can trigger nonobese impaired glucose tolerance caused by insulin-secretion defect (Hattori et al. 2021). High-fructose corn syrup was shown to not only trigger impaired glucose tolerance, but it also further increase blood triglyceride levels (Mock et al. 2017), fasting blood glucose (Takata et al. 2019), adipose tissue hypertrophy, and body weight (Sheludiakova et al. 2012; Shintani et al. 2017). By contrast, several studies by Tsilas et al. (2017) and Sadowska and Rygielska (2019) found that consumption of fructose-containing sugar is not associated with the development of Type 2 diabetes. *Pdx1*, a transcriptional factor, is essential for the improvement of insulin replication and secretion of β-cells (Melloul et al. 2002; Kulkarni et al. 2004). Phosphorylation of *Pdx1* in β-cells induces diabetes and insulin-secretion disorders (Ahlgren et al. 1998; Gao et al. 2014). Some studies by Aughsteen et al. (2005) and Madole et al. (2016) reported that individuals with diabetes have relatively low serum pancreatic amylase levels.

Type 2 diabetes is characterized by insulin resistance and ultimately leads to the failure of insulin secretion, which is associated with the reduced pancreatic β-cell mass or dysfunction of pancreatic islet cells. In pancreatic β cells, administration of fructose failed to lead to insulin secretion, and constant exposure caused the increased reactivity of pancreatic β cells to glucose (Bartley et al. 2019). Intakes of fructose accelerated dysfunction of islets through induction of oxidative stress and islet inflammation (Cummings et al. 2010). Although the previous study suggests that fructose may act directly on the pancreas, further studies are warranted to evaluate whether circulating fructose after hepatic and intestinal clearance is sufficiently high to affect the pancreas *in vivo* (Jung et al. 2022).

A study by Corte et al. (2021) evaluated the prospective association of dietary sugar consumption in adolescence with biomarkers of inflammation and insulin sensitivity in young adulthood. The researchers did not identify a relationship between urinary or dietary sugars and the adult pro-inflammatory score, which includes adiponectin, chemerin, leptin, interleukin-18 (IL-18), IL-6, and C-reactive protein (CRP). Additionally, the study found no association between dietary sugar consumption during adolescence and insulin sensitivity in adulthood. However, moderate fructose consumption showed a beneficial association with fasting insulin levels and the homeostasis model assessment of insulin sensitivity (HOMA2-S%) (Corte et al. 2021). Fructose intake leads to smaller insulin excursions due to its inability to stimulate insulin secretion from pancreatic beta cells. The evidence is further supported by a meta-analysis of randomized trials, in which iso-energetic replacements of sucrose and glucose with fructose led to a reduction of insulin levels (Wu et al. 2004). In general, the human diet seldom encounters fructose as a single nutrient. A meta-analysis revealed that intakes of small doses of fructose in iso-energetic exchange enhanced fasting blood glucose and HbA1c but had no effect on insulin resistance (Noronha et al. 2018).

The available data imply that high-carbohydrate diets induce oxidative stress by increasing inflammatory markers and augmenting the inflammatory response. The progression and development of diabetes mellitus are linked to insulin resistance and β cell dysfunction, and this phenomenon is commonly associated with obesity. Collectively, more randomized clinical trials are required to elucidate the overall long-term effects of dietary intervention.

References

Adedeji TG, Abosede CO, Dareowolabi BO (2022) A high carbohydrate and soda diet influences metabolic variables in Wistar rats. Life Sci 291:120295

Ahlgren U, Jonsson J, Jonsson L et al (1998) Beta-cell-specific inactivation of the mouse Ipf1/Pdx1 gene results in loss of the beta -cell phenotype and maturity onset diabetes. Genes Dev 12:1763–1768

Alzamendi A, Giovambattista A, Raschia A et al (2009) Fructose-rich diet-induced abdominal adipose tissue endocrine dysfunction in normal male rats. Endocrine 35:227–232

Arias-Chávez DJ, Mailloux-Salinas P, Altamirano J et al (2022) Consumption of combined fructose and sucrose diet exacerbates oxidative stress, hypertrophy and CaMKIIδ oxidation in hearts from rats with metabolic syndrome. Mol Cell Biochem 477:1309–1320

Aughsteen AA, Abu-Umair MS, Mahmoud AS (2005) Biochemical analysis of serum pancreatic amylase and lipase enzymes in patients with type 1 and type 2 diabetes mellitus. Saudi Med J 26:73–77

Bartley C, Brun T, Oberhauser L et al (2019) Chronic fructose renders pancreatic β-cells hyperresponsive to glucose-stimulated insulin secretion through extracellular ATP signaling. Am J Physiol Endocrinol Metab 317:E25–E41

Brownlee M (2001) Biochemistry and molecular cell biology of diabetic complications. Nature 414:813–820

Burén J, Liu H-X, Lauritz J et al (2003) High glucose and insulin in combination cause insulin receptor substrate-1 and -2 depletion and protein kinase B desensitisation in primary cultured rat adipocytes: possible implications for insulin resistance in type 2 diabetes. Eur J Endocrinol 148:157–167

Castro MC, Massa ML, Del Zotto H et al (2011) Rat liver uncoupling protein 2: changes induced by a fructose-rich diet. Life Sci 89:609–614

Castro MC, Francini F, Schinella G et al (2012) Apocynin administration prevents the changes induced by a fructoserich diet on rat liver metabolism and the antioxidant system. Clin Sci 123:681–692

Castro MC, Francini F, Gagliardino JJ et al (2014) Lipoic acid prevents fructose-induced changes in liver carbohydrate metabolism: role of oxidative stress. Biochim Biophys Acta 1840:1145–1151

Castro MC, Massa ML, Arbeláez LG et al (2015) Fructose-induced inflammation, insulin resistance and oxidative stress: a liver pathological triad effectively disrupted by lipoic acid. Life Sci 137:1–6

Catena C, Cavarape A, Novello M et al (2003) Insulin receptors and renal sodium handling in hypertensive fructose-fed rats. Kidney Int 64:2163–2171

Chen C, Cohrs CM, Stertmann J, Bozsak R, Speier S (2017) Human beta cell mass and function in diabetes: recent advances in knowledge and technologies to understand disease pathogenesis. Mol Metab 6:943–957

Corte KAD, Penczynski K, Kuhnle G et al (2021) The prospective association of dietary sugar intake in adolescence with risk markers of type 2 diabetes in young adulthood. Front Nutr 7:615684

Cummings BP, Stanhope KL, Graham JL et al (2010) Dietary fructose accelerates the development of diabetes in UCD-T2DM rats: amelioration by the antioxidant, α-lipoic acid. Am J Physiol Regul Integr Comp Physiol 298:R1343–R1350

de Koning L, Malik VS, Kellogg MD et al (2012) Sweetened beverage consumption, incident coronary heart disease, and biomarkers of risk in men. Circulation 125:1735–1741

DiNicolantonio JJ, O'Keefe JH, Lucan SC (2015) Added fructose: a principle driver of type 2 diabetes mellitus and its consequences. Mayo Clin Proc 90:372–381

Evans RA, Frese M, Romero J et al (2017) Fructose replacement of glucose or sucrose in food or beverages lowers postprandial glucose and insulin without raising triglycerides: a systematic review and meta-analysis. Am J Clin Nutr 106:506–518

Francini F, Castro MC, Schinella G et al (2010) Changes induced by a fructose-rich diet on hepatic metabolism and the antioxidant system. Life Sci 86:965–971

Gao T, McKenna B, Li C et al (2014) Pdx1 maintains β cell identity and function by repressing an α-cell program. Cell Metab 19:259–271

Godoy JR, Funke M, Ackermann W et al (2011) Redox atlas of the mouse: immunohistochemical detection of glutaredoxin-, peroxiredoxin-, and thioredoxin-family proteins in various tissues of the laboratory mouse. Biochim. Biophys. Acta Gen. Subj. 1810:2–92

Goran MI, Ulijaszek SJ, Ventura EE (2013) High fructose corn syrup and diabetes prevalence: a global perspective. Glob Public Health 8:55–64

Hanover LM, White JS (1993) Manufacturing, composition, and applications of fructose. Am J Clin Nutr 58:724S–732S

Hattori H, Hanai Y, Oshima Y et al (2021) Excessive intake of high-fructose corn syrup drinks induces impaired glucose tolerance. Biomedicines 9:541

Henriksen EJ, Diamond-Stanic MK, Marchionne EM (2011) Oxidative stress and the etiology of insulin resistance and type 2 diabetes. Free Radic Biol Med 51:993–999

Hu FB, Malik VS (2010) Sugar-sweetened beverages and risk of obesity and type 2 diabetes: epidemiologic evidence. Physiol Behav 100:47–54

Hu EA, Pan A, Malik V et al (2012) White rice consumption and risk of type 2 diabetes: meta-analysis and systematic review. BMJ 344:e1454

Jung S, Bae H, Song W-S et al (2022) Dietary fructose and fructose-induced pathologies. Annu Rev Nutr 42:45–66

Kulkarni RN, Jhala US, Winnay JN et al (2004) PDX-1 haploinsufficiency limits the compensatory islet hyperplasia that occurs in response to insulin resistance. J Clin Invest 114:828–836

Lal MK, Singh B, Sharma S et al (2021) Glycemic index of starchy crops and factors affecting its digestibility: a review. Trends Food Sci Technol 111:741–755

Livesey G, Taylor R (2008) Fructose consumption and consequences for glycation, plasma triacylglycerol, and body weight: meta-analyses and meta-regression models of intervention studies. Am J Clin Nutr 88:1419–1437

Madole MB, Iyer CM, Madivalar MT et al (2016) Evaluation of biochemical markers serum amylase and serum lipase for the assessment of pancreatic exocrine function in diabetes mellitus. J Clin Diagn Res 10:BC01–BC04

Malik VS, Popkin BM, Bray GA et al (2010) Sugar-sweetened beverages and risk of metabolic syndrome and type 2 diabetes: a meta-analysis. Diabetes Care 33:2477–2483

Mehmeti I, Gurgul-Convey E, Lenzen S et al (2011) Induction of the intrinsic apoptosis pathway in insulin-secreting cells is dependent on oxidative damage of mitochondria but independent of caspase-12 activation. Biochim et Biophys Acta (BBA)–Mol Cell Res 1813:1827–1835

Melloul D, Marshak S, Cerasi E (2002) Regulation of insulin gene transcription. Diabetologia 45:309–326

Mock K, Lateef S, Benedito VA et al (2017) High-fructose corn syrup-55 consumption alters hepatic lipid metabolism and promotes triglyceride accumulation. J Nutr Biochem 39:32–39

Nanri A, Mizoue T, Noda M et al (2010) Rice intake and type 2 diabetes in Japanese men and women: the Japan public health center-based prospective study. Am J Clin Nutr 92:1468–1477

Noronha JC, Braunstein CR, Blanco Mejia S et al (2018) The effect of small doses of fructose and its epimers on glycemic control: a systematic review and meta-analysis of controlled feeding trials. Nutrients 10:1805

O'Connor L, Imamura F, Lentjes MA et al (2015) Prospective associations and population impact of sweet beverage intake and type 2 diabetes, and effects of substitutions with alternative beverages. Diabetologia 58:1474–1483

Prentki M, Matschinsky FM, Madiraju SRM (2013) Metabolic signaling in fuel-induced insulin secretion. Cell Metab 18:162–185

Radhika G, Van Dam RM, Sudha V et al (2009) Refined grain consumption and the metabolic syndrome in urban Asian Indians (Chennai urban rural epidemiology study 57). Metabolism 58:675–681

Roma LP, Jonas J-C (2020) Nutrient metabolism, subcellular redox state, and oxidative stress in pancreatic islets and β-cells. J Mol Biol 432:1461–1493

Sadowska J, Rygielska M (2019) The effect of high fructose corn syrup on the plasma insulin and leptin concentration, body weight gain and fat accumulation in rat. Adv Clin Exp Med 28:879–884

Sakai K, Matsumoto K, Nishikawa T et al (2003) Mitochondrial reactive oxygen species reduce insulin secretion by pancreatic β-cells. Biochem Biophys Res Commun 300:216–222

Scharfmann R, Rachdi L, Ravassard P (2013) Concise review: in search of unlimited sources of functional human pancreatic beta cells. Stem Cells Transl Med 2:61–67

Schulze MB, Manson JE, Ludwig DS et al (2004) Sugar-sweetened beverages, weight gain, and incidence of type 2 diabetes in young and middle-aged women. JAMA 292:927–934

Sheludiakova A, Rooney K, Boakes RA (2012) Metabolic and behavioural effects of sucrose and fructose/glucose drinks in the rat. Eur J Nutr 51:445–454

Shintani T, Yamada T, Hayashi N et al (2017) Rare sugar syrup containing d-Allulose but not high-fructose corn syrup maintains glucose tolerance and insulin sensitivity partly via hepatic glucokinase translocation in Wistar rats. J Agric Food Chem 65:2888–2894

Song S, Lee JE, Song WO et al (2014) Carbohydrate intake and refined-grain consumption are associated with metabolic syndrome in the Korean adult population. J Acad Nutr Dietetics 114:54–62

Stanhope KL, Bremer AA, Medici V et al (2011) Consumption of fructose and high fructose corn syrup increase postprandial triglycerides, LDL-cholesterol, and apolipoprotein-B in young men and women. J Clin Endocrinol Metab 96:E1596–E1605

Takasaki Y (1966) Studies on sugar-isomerizing enzyme. Agric Biol Chem 30:1247–1253

Takata T, Sakasai-Sakai A, Takino J-I et al (2019) Evidence for toxic advanced glycation end-products generated in the normal rat liver. Nutrients 11:1612

Tan BL, Norhaizan ME (2021) The role of antioxidants in longevity and age-related diseases. In: Tan BL, Norhaizan ME (eds) Chapter 3 age-related oxidative stress-induced redox imbalance. Springer Nature, Cham, pp 27–37

Teff KL, Elliott SS, Tschöp M et al (2004) Dietary fructose reduces circulating insulin and leptin, attenuates postprandial suppression of ghrelin, and increases triglycerides in women. J Clin Endocrinol Metab 89:2963–2972

Teff KL, Grudziak J, Townsend RR et al (2009) Endocrine and metabolic effects of consuming fructose-and glucose-sweetened beverages with meals in obese men and women: influence of insulin resistance on plasma triglyceride responses. J Clin Endocrinol Metab 94:1562–1569

Teodoro JS, Duarte FV, Gomes AP et al (2013) Berberine reverts hepatic mitochondrial dysfunction in high-fat fed rats: a possible role for SirT3 activation. Mitochondrion 13:637–646

Thirunavukkarasu V, Anitha Nandhini AT, Anuradha CV (2004) Effect of α-lipoic acid on lipid profile in rats fed a high-fructose diet. Exp Diabesity Res 5:195–200

Tsilas CS, de Souza RJ, Mejia SB et al (2017) Relation of total sugars, fructose and sucrose with incident type 2 diabetes: a systematic review and meta-analysis of prospective cohort studies. Can Med Assoc J 189:E711–E720

Utzschneider KM, Kahn SE (2006) The role of insulin resistance in nonalcoholic fatty liver disease. J Clin Endocrinol Metab 91:4753–4761

Wang DD, Sievenpiper JL, de Souza RJ et al (2014) Effect of fructose on postprandial triglycerides: a systematic review and meta-analysis of controlled feeding trials. Atherosclerosis 232:125–133

Wehinger S, Ortiz R, Díaz MI et al (2015) Phosphorylation of caveolin-1 on tyrosine-14 induced by ROS enhances palmitate-induced death of beta-pancreatic cells. Biochim et Biophys Acta (BBA)—Mol Basis Dis 1852:693–708

White JS (2013) Challenging the fructose hypothesis: new perspectives on fructose consumption and metabolism. Oxford University Press, Oxford

Wu T, Giovannucci E, Pischon T et al (2004) Fructose, glycemic load, and quantity and quality of carbohydrate in relation to plasma C-peptide concentrations in US women. Am J Clin Nutr 80:1043–1049

Wu J, Luo X, Thangthaeng N et al (2017) Pancreatic mitochondrial complex I exhibits aberrant hyperactivity in diabetes. Biochem Biophys Rep 11:119–129

Zafar MI, Mills KE, Zheng J et al (2019) Low-glycemic index diets as an intervention for diabetes: a systematic review and meta-analysis. Am J Clin Nutr 110:891–902

Chapter 6
High Animal-Based Proteins and Cancer

6.1 Protein

Protein is comprised of amino acids essential for human health at all ages and is commonly utilized in the food industry to produce a broad spectrum of healthy diets for nutritional demands. Dietary protein is the main nitrogen source, in which amino acid serves as a building block for body tissues and modulates physiological enzymes vital in regulating biological and chemical reactions. Indeed, protein is commonly utilized as a surface-active agent in the food industry due to its amphiphilic nature (Akharume et al. 2021). Despite animal protein being a good source of protein for food production, it has drawn a great deal of attention to environmental issues, for instance, increased greenhouse gas emissions during the production of meat (Qin et al. 2022). Moreover, long-term red meat intake can increase the development of chronic diseases including cancer (Ahnen et al. 2019; Hertzler et al. 2020).

Protein quality is commonly associated with its composition of essential amino acids and its digestibility in the human body after consumption. Animl proteins including milk, eggs, and meat, contain complete amino acids, known as "complete protein packages" (Shams-White et al. 2018). Animal protein is comprised of essential amino acids including valine, tryptophan, threonine, phenylalanine, methionine, lysine, leucine, isoleucine, and histidine (Nosenko 2017). Protein digestibility is the fraction of ingested amino acids that can be made available for utilization by the body after absorption and digestion. Animal protein contains more than 95% digestibility, imply that most animal protein can be used after digestion (Harwatt 2019; Päivärinta et al. 2020).

6.2 Meat and Cancer Risk

Meat consists of a crucial fraction of a normal diet and is composed of 40% of daily protein, 15% of energy intake, and 20% of daily fat (Food and Agriculture Organization of the United Nations Statistics Division 2010). Meat is high in saturated fatty acids and dietary protein. Excessive consumption of processed meat is likely to increase the risk of cancer (Nouri-Majd et al. 2022). Processed and red meat contains polycyclic aromatic hydrocarbons (PAHs), N-nitroso compounds (NOCs), heterocyclic amines (HCAs), and heme iron that are generated by prolonged or high-temperature cooking (Domingo and Nadal 2017; Sasso and Latella 2018). An animal study demonstrated that these compounds were carcinogenic (Odashima 1980). The data from the meta-analysis and systematic review included 25 prospective studies demonstrated that increased intake of processed meat and total meat might be linked to a greater risk of prostate cancer (Nouri-Majd et al. 2022). The study further demonstrated that an increment of 50 g of processed meat per day may link to a 4% greater risk of total prostate cancer (Nouri-Majd et al. 2022). Sinha et al. (2009) and Rodriguez et al. (2006) further revealed that processed and red meat was linked to the risk of prostate cancer. Data from meta-analysis and systematic review of prospective studies revealed that intake of red meat was significantly linked to a greater hepatocellular carcinoma, lung cancer, colorectal cancer, endometrial cancer, and breast cancer risk (Farvid et al. 2021). Further, the study indicates that processed meat was significantly linked to a 12% greater lung cancer risk, 22% greater rectal cancer risk, 21% greater colon cancer risk, 18% greater colorectal cancer risk, and 6% greater breast cancer risk (Farvid et al. 2021). This finding reveals that high intake of red meat was positively associated with hepatocellular carcinoma, lung cancer, colorectal cancer, breast cancer, and endometrial cancer risk, and high intakes of processed meat was positively linked to lung, rectal, colon, colorectal, and breast risk (Farvid et al. 2021). However, meta-analyses of prospective cohort studies failed to show any relationship between processed or red meat intakes and prostate cancer risk (Alexander et al. 2010; Bylsma and Alexander 2015), with a weak positive relationship reported between total prostate cancer risk and processed meat intake (Bylsma and Alexander 2015).

A meta-analysis analyzed of 32 prospective cohort studies included 31 meta-analysis and 32 prospective cohort studies revealed that consumption of animal protein was not significantly related to cancer mortality. Likewise, the study also found that intake of animal protein was not associated with cardiovascular disease risk (Naghshi et al. 2020). Intriguingly, the study showed that an additional 3% energy from plant proteins daily was linked to a 5% decreased risk of death from all causes, suggesting that substituting foods high in animal protein with plant protein may link to longevity (Naghshi et al. 2020). Evidence from a population-based study demonstrated that high intakes of animal-derived proteins were linked to a greater risk of mortality in community-dwelling men aged ≥70 years. Nonetheless, the substitution of animal protein with plant-derived protein decreased the mortality risk (Das et al. 2022). Mehta et al. (2020) explored the impacts of red and processed meats on the development of colorectal cancer in U.S. women aged 35–74 years old. The data showed that processed meat intake such as sausages and bacon was linked to a high risk of colorectal cancer. In the context of cooking methods, grilled/barbequed steaks and hamburgers were related to the elevated risk of colorectal cancer in women (Mehta et al. 2020). Niedermaier et al. (2023) further revealed that the elimination of processed meat intake may decrease the burden of colorectal cancer about 205,000 cases in Germany (9.6%) in 2020–2050, 1/3 among females (60,000), and 2/3 in males (145,000). A macro-simulation approach further demonstrated that decreased mean intakes of red and processed meat by one or two servings (22 or 11 g per day) would be expected to decrease colorectal cancer case numbers by 140,000 (6.5%) and 68,000 (3.1%), respectively. These data imply that a decrease in processed and red meat consumption may substantially reduce colorectal cancer incidence in Germany (Niedermaier et al. 2023).

6.3 Fish and Cancer Risk

Fish is a predominant component of the Mediterranean diet, and its intake is often actively encouraged as it contains fatty acids, high-quality protein, and essential micronutrients (minerals and vitamins). Indeed, fish is the major dietary source of long-chain omega-3 polyunsaturated fatty acids (ω-3 PUFA), including eicosapentaenoic acid (EPA) and docosahexaenoic acid (DHA), which exerts immunomodulatory and anti-inflammatory properties (Tan et al. 2018). Research evidence suggests that fish oil containing ω-3 PUFA suppresses colorectal carcinogenesis via modulation of several pathways (Hou et al. 2016; Irún et al. 2019). Likewise, the finding of meta-analysis further demonstrated that intake of ω-3 PUFA is inversely linked to colorectal cancer risk (Kim and Kim 2020). Data from the meta-analysis included 25 prospective epidemiological studies with 25,777 colorectal cancer cases from inception to November 2020 showed that consumption of fish significantly decreased the risk of colorectal cancer.

6.4 Mechanism of Cancer Triggered by Red/Processed Meat

The mechanisms that implicate the risk of prostate cancer and red or processed meat intake are complex and involve several potential modes of action. For instance, heme iron in processed and red meat and N-nitroso compounds (NOCs) in processed meat are regarded as DNA-damaging factors (Bellamri and Turesky 2019). In general, heme iron is carried by hemoglobin or directly through the bloodstream in the body, which can catalyze the oxidative reactions that may lead to lipid, protein, and DNA oxidations in several organs including the prostate (Bellamri and Turesky 2019). NOCs in processed meat are produced through the reaction between nitrates or nitrites and amides or amines (Johnson 2017), and the presence of NOCs in processed meat may enhance the cancer risk (Domingo and Nadal 2017). Heterocyclic amines (HCAs) and polycyclic aromatic hydrocarbons (PAHs) in cooked foods, particularly in meat, have been linked to an increased risk of several cancers (Ali et al. 2019). HCAs are mutagenic compounds believed to play a significant role in the development of human cancers. Notably, research has shown that 2-Amino-1-methyl-6-phenylimiazo[4,5-b]pyridine (PhIP) forms DNA adducts in the human prostate, which can lead to abnormal prostate cells (Bellamri et al. 2018). Additionally, excessive fat intake from meat can elevate hormone production, such as estrogens, which may further increase the risk of hormone-related cancers, including prostate and breast cancer (Oczkowski et al. 2021).

Moreover, the consumption of red meat has emerged as a significant risk factor for colorectal cancer. Evidence suggests that heme iron, a key component of red meat, may contribute to colorectal carcinogenesis. Dietary heme catalyzes lipid peroxidation and stimulates the reactive aldehydes, as measured using thiobarbituric acid reactive substance (TBARS). Elevation of heme-induced TBARS levels in fecal water was linked to high cytotoxicity and luminal injury when fecal water is applied to cultured colonocytes (Seiwert et al. 2020). An early study showed that dietary heme suppresses apoptosis and downregulates caspase-3 activity in the colon mucosa (de Vogel et al. 2008). Red meat such as lamb and beef is characterized by its high myoglobin content and shows a higher heme iron level compared to white meat, for instance, chicken (Bak et al. 2019). Research evidence showed that intake of processed and red meat accounts for 1.18 and 1.77% of colorectal cancer mortality worldwide, respectively. Intriguingly, the death risk attributed to red meat consumption has increased linearly in recent decades, while processed meat showed a linear decrease (Mattiuzzi and Lippi 2020).

Dietary heme leads a microbial dysbiosis and impairs the intestinal barrier and therefore exposing the epithelium to enterobacteria, and subsequently to bacterial lipopolysaccharides (LPS). Seiwert et al. (2020) suggested that heme iron, either bound or free as a prosthetic group to myoglobin or hemoglobin, promotes the formation of colorectal cancer. Dietary heme possesses pro-tumorigenic activity in the colorectum on multiple layers and thus favors sporadic colorectal cancer formation, which occurs predominantly through the adenoma-carcinoma sequence (Seiwert et al. 2020). Heme iron promotes different DNA damaging agents such as N-nitroso compounds (NOC), lipid peroxidation end-products, and reactive oxygen species (ROS).

Evidence from prospective epidemiological studies suggested that fish intakes may decrease colorectal cancer risk (Caini et al. 2022). Fish or fish oil protects against colorectal carcinogenesis via several mechanisms. Omega-3 PUFA modulates eicosanoid metabolism by suppressing the production of prostaglandin E2 (PGE_2) levels, in which eicosapentaenoic acid (EPA) can serve as a substrate for cyclooxygenase (COXs) to synthesize unique 3-series prostaglandin compounds, such as PGE_3 (Yang et al. 2014). Furthermore, ω-3 PUFA does not stimulate the luminal concentration of secondary bile acids and decreases liver and colon activity of tyrosine-specific protein kinase (TPK) and ornithine decarboxylase (ODC), which all are implicated in colon carcinogenesis (Reddy 2004). The positive epigenetic effects have also been demonstrated along with the interaction of ω-3 PUFA with transcription factors and nuclear receptors, and therefore lead to an alteration of apoptosis, lipid metabolism, and proliferation of cancer cells (Hou et al. 2016). Importantly, ω-3 PUFA was also found to be linked to higher intestinal microbial diversity, enhancing host immune function and ultimately halting colorectal cancer development (Song and Chan 2019; Piazzi et al. 2019).

Consumption of processed meat may be linked to an elevated risk of advanced and total prostate cancer (Nouri-Majd et al. 2022). In this regard, it seems that replacing processed and red meats should be shifted toward healthier animal protein alternatives, for instance, dairy products and white meat. The available research evidence demonstrated that fish consumption may prevent colorectal cancer. Therefore, the possible risks of consuming processed meat could be stated on the nutrition label. The potential implications of red and processed meat and fish on cancer are worth further investigation in comparative randomized clinical trials.

References

Ahnen RT, Jonnalagadda SS, Slavin JL (2019) Role of plant protein in nutrition, wellness, and health. Nutr Rev 77:735–747

Akharume FU, Aluko RE, Adedeji AA (2021) Modification of plant proteins for improved functionality: a review. Compr Rev Food Sci Food Saf 20:198–224

Alexander DD, Mink PJ, Cushing CA et al (2010) A review and meta-analysis of prospective studies of red and processed meat intake and prostate cancer. Nutr J 9:50

Ali A, Waly MI, Devarajan S (2019) Impact of processing meat on the formation of heterocyclic amines and risk of cancer. In: Biogenic amines in food. Royal Society of Chemistry, Muscat, pp 187–211

Bak KH, Bolumar T, Karlsson AH et al (2019) Effect of high pressure treatment on the color of fresh and processed meats: a review. Crit Rev Food Sci Nutr 59:228–252

Bellamri M, Turesky RJ (2019) Dietary carcinogens and DNA adducts in prostate cancer. Adv Exp Med Biol 1210:29–55

Bellamri M, Xiao S, Murugan P et al (2018) Metabolic activation of the cooked meat carcinogen 2-amino-1-methyl-6-phenylimidazo [4, 5-b] pyridine in human prostate. Toxicol Sci 163:543–556

Bylsma LC, Alexander DD (2015) A review and meta-analysis of prospective studies of red and processed meat, meat cooking methods, heme iron, heterocyclic amines and prostate cancer. Nutr J 14:125

Caini S, Chioccioli S, Pastore E et al (2022) Fish consumption and colorectal cancer risk: meta-analysis of prospective epidemiological studies and review of evidence from animal studies. Cancers 14:640

Das A, Cumming R, Naganathan V et al (2022) Associations between dietary intake of total protein and sources of protein (plant vs. animal) and risk of all-cause and cause-specific mortality in older Australian men: the Concord health and ageing in men project. J Hum Nutr Diet 35:845–860

de Vogel J, van Eck WB, Sesink ALA et al (2008) Dietary heme injures surface epithelium resulting in hyperproliferation, inhibition of apoptosis and crypt hyperplasia in rat colon. Carcinogenesis 29:398–403

Domingo JL, Nadal M (2017) Carcinogenicity of consumption of red meat and processed meat: a review of scientific news since the IARC decision. Food Chem Toxicol 105:256–261

Farvid MS, Sidahmed E, Spence ND et al (2021) Consumption of red meat and processed meat and cancer incidence: a systematic review and meta-analysis of prospective studies. Eur J Epidemiol 36:937–951

Food and Agriculture Organization of the United Nations Statistics Division (2010) Food balance sheets millennium issue 1999–2001 special charts. http://www.fao.org/economic/ess/food-balance-sheets-millennium-issue-1999-2001-special-charts/en/

Harwatt H (2019) Including animal to plant protein shifts in climate change mitigation policy: a proposed three-step strategy. Clim Pol 19:533–541

Hertzler SR, Lieblein-Boff JC, Weiler M et al (2020) Plant proteins: assessing their nutritional quality and effects on health and physical function. Nutrients 12:3704

Hou TY, Davidson LA, Kim E et al (2016) Nutrient-gene interaction in colon cancer, from the membrane to cellular physiology. Annu Rev Nutr 36:543–570

Irún P, Lanas A, Piazuelo E (2019) Omega-3 polyunsaturated fatty acids and their bioactive metabolites in gastrointestinal malignancies related to unresolved inflammation. A review. Front Pharmacol 10:852

Johnson IT (2017) The cancer risk related to meat and meat products. Br Med Bull 121:73–81

Kim Y, Kim J (2020) Intake or blood levels of n-3 polyunsaturated fatty acids and risk of colorectal cancer: a systematic review and meta-analysis of prospective studies. Cancer Epidemiol Biomarkers Prev 29:288–299

Mattiuzzi C, Lippi G (2020) Epidemiologic burden of red and processed meat intake on colorectal cancer mortality. Nutr Cancer 73:562–567

Mehta SS, Arroyave WD, Lunn RM et al (2020) A prospective analysis of red and processed meat consumption and risk of colorectal cancer in women. Cancer Epidemiol Biomarkers Prev 29:141–150

Naghshi S, Sadeghi O, Willett WC et al (2020) Dietary intake of total, animal, and plant proteins and risk of all cause, cardiovascular, and cancer mortality: systematic review and dose-response meta-analysis of prospective cohort studies. BMJ 370:m2412

Niedermaier T, Gredner T, Hoffmeister M et al (2023) Impact of reducing intake of red and processed meat on colorectal cancer incidence in Germany 2020 to 2050—a simulation study. Nutrients 15:1020

Nosenko T (2017) Comparison of biological value and technological properties of oil seed proteins. Ukr Food J 6:226–238

Nouri-Majd S, Salari-Moghaddam A, Aminianfar A et al (2022) Association between red and processed meat consumption and risk of prostate cancer: a systematic review and meta-analysis. Front Nutr 9:801722

Oczkowski M, Dziendzikowska K, Pasternak-Winiarska A et al (2021) Dietary factors and prostate cancer development, progression, and reduction. Nutrients 13:496

Odashima S (1980) Overview: N-nitroso compounds as carcinogens for experimental animals and man. Oncology 37:282–286

Päivärinta E, Itkonen ST, Pellinen T et al (2020) Replacing animal-based proteins with plant-based proteins changes the composition of a whole nordic diet-a randomised clinical trial in healthy Finnish adults. Nutrients 12:943

Piazzi G, Prossomariti A, Baldassarre M et al (2019) A Mediterranean diet mix has chemopreventive effects in a murine model of colorectal cancer modulating apoptosis and the gut microbiota. Front Oncol 9:140

Qin P, Wang T, Luo Y (2022) A review on plant-based proteins from soybean: health benefits and soy product development. J Agric Food Res 7:100265

Reddy BS (2004) Studies with the azoxymethane-rat preclinical model for assessing colon tumor development and chemoprevention. Environ Mol Mutagen 44:26–35

Rodriguez C, McCullough ML, Mondul AM et al (2006) Meat consumption among black and White men and risk of prostate cancer in the cancer prevention study II nutrition cohort. Cancer Epidemiol Biomarkers Prev 15:211–216

Sasso A, Latella G (2018) Role of heme iron in the association between red meat consumption and colorectal cancer. Nutr Cancer 70:1173–1183

Seiwert N, Heylmann D, Hasselwander S et al (2020) Mechanism of colorectal carcinogenesis triggered by heme iron from red meat. Biochim et Biophys Acta (BBA) Rev Cancer 1873:188334

Shams-White MM, Chung M, Fu Z et al (2018) Animal versus plant protein and adult bone health: a systematic review and meta-analysis from the National Osteoporosis Foundation. PLoS One 13:e0192459

Sinha R, Park Y, Graubard BI et al (2009) Meat and meat-related compounds and risk of prostate cancer in a large prospective cohort study in the United States. Am J Epidemiol 170:1165–1177

Song M, Chan AT (2019) Environmental factors, gut microbiota, and colorectal cancer prevention. Clin Gastroenterol Hepatol 17:275–289

Tan BL, Norhaizan ME, Liew W-P-P (2018) Nutrients and oxidative stress: Friend or foe. Oxid Med Cell Longev Volume 2018, Article ID 9719584, p 24

Yang P, Jiang Y, Fischer SM (2014) Prostaglandin E3 metabolism and cancer. Cancer Lett 348:1–11

Chapter 7
Excessive Consumption of Fats and Cardiovascular Disease

Achieving sustained and vital lifestyle changes required consistent and clear public health concerns. Nonetheless, the general public has been bombarded with conflicting and confusing recommendations on diet. This could be attributed to the presumption that the relationship between macronutrients and health outcomes is linear across different intakes irrespective of the level of consumption of total energy and other macronutrients (Ho et al. 2020).

In general, the dietary recommendation has included sugar, carbohydrate, saturated fat, and fat (FAO 2018). Emerging research evidence indicates that decreased consumption of saturated fat can reduce cardiovascular events (Mozaffarian et al. 2010). Despite the favorable effect of reduction of saturated fat on cardiovascular events was reported, not all data demonstrated such an association. Data from the meta-analyses of prospective cohort studies failed to show any associations (Siri-Tarino et al. 2010). This historical advice was challenged by several meta-analyses of prospective studies (Siri-Tarino et al. 2010; de Souza et al. 2015), including the World Health Organization (WHO 2018) and UK Scientific Advisory Committee on Nutrition (SACN) (SACN 2019), in which consumption of saturated fat is not linked to the cardiovascular mortality. Similarly, a study by SACN also showed an inconsistency between prospective cohort studies and randomized controlled trials on the relationship between saturated fat consumption and cardiovascular events (such as peripheral vascular disease, cerebrovascular disease, and ischaemic heart disease) (SACN 2019).

The role of lipids as causal factors for CVD is well established. Dietary saturated fats (SFA) including coconut oil, palm oil, poultry, pork, lamb, beef, cheese, butter, and milk increase high-density lipoprotein cholesterol (HDL-C) and low-density lipoprotein cholesterol (LDL-C). The elevation of LDL-C could be attributed to an increase in LDL generation secondary to a reduction in hepatic LDL receptors and a reduction of hepatic LDL clearance. Monounsaturated fatty acids (MUFA) can be found in seeds and nuts, peanut butter, avocados, sesame, safflower, peanut, canola, and olive oil, whereas soybeans, tofu, some seeds and nuts, and sunflower, corn, and soybean oil are rich in polyunsaturated fatty acids (PUFA) (Koneru et al. 2023). The previous study showed that both PUFA and MUFA can lower LDL-C by elevating hepatic LDL receptor activity. Dietary cholesterol is found in butter, cheese, poultry, pork, beef, shrimp, and egg yolks and increases LDL-C but the effect is modest and varied by individuals from 15–25%. Dietary cholesterol increases LDL production, reduces clearance, and decreases hepatic LDL receptor activity.

7.1 Cardiovascular Disease

CVD including heart disease is the predominant cause of mortality worldwide. According to the World Health Organization (2024), approximately 17.9 million lives are killed due to CVD yearly. More than four out of five CVD deaths are caused by heart attacks and strokes, in one-third of these deaths occurred prematurely in individuals under 70 years old (World Health Organization 2024). Diabetes, obesity, high blood pressure, reduced HDL-C, increased LDL-C, hypertriglyceridemia, and high cholesterol are preventable risk factors for CVD (Nowbar et al. 2019). Unhealthy lifestyles including dietary habits are thought to play a critical role in the development of heart disease (Tan et al. 2018b).

Nutrition affects atherosclerosis was first reported by Ignatowski (1908), in which diets high in animal proteins (eggs, meat, and milk) fed to rabbits led to intimal lesions with large clear cells known as foam cell accumulation in the aorta. A study by Anitschkow showed that rabbits fed with a high-cholesterol diet caused aortic atherosclerosis similar to in humans (Steinberg 2004). The study further proposed a causal role of cholesterol in atherosclerosis, which remains a consensus (Steinberg 2004). Hence, cholesterol was isolated in human atherosclerotic plaques (Ahrens Jr et al. 1957). In general, the underlying cause of CVD is atherosclerosis, a chronic inflammation of the arteries, which has developed in response to the underlying risk factors in recent decades (Libby 2021; Fan and Watanabe 2022).

Emerging evidence highlights the effects of diet on CVD risk and this literature is often controversial and conflicting. Yet, the National Health Institution has traditionally recommended decreasing the consumption of dietary fat for CVD prevention (Nations FaAOotU 2010). Similarly, the consumption of trans fat has been reported to be related to health outcomes, and thereby it is recommended to decrease its intake to a minimum (Michas et al. 2014). There are several limitations to concluding randomized controlled trials including (1) accuracy of the methods utilized to evaluate lipid levels; (2) dietary composition or differences in the types of diet; (3) adherence to the study diet; (4) variation in the baseline diets; (5) study design; (6) types of individuals studied; (7) heterogeneity in study settings. In addition, the lipid response of an individual to dietary manipulations can be varied. The genetic differences in this response are usually underestimated by providers and patients. For instance, individuals with an apo E4 allele are more likely to reduce LDL-C in response to a reduction in cholesterol and dietary fat compared to respondents carrying apo E2 or apo E3 alleles (Ordovas et al. 1995). Polymorphisms in other genes have also been demonstrated to mediate the lipid response to dietary manipulations (Ordovas et al. 1995; Vazquez-Vidal et al. 2019).

7.2   Dietary Saturated Fatty Acids

Saturated fatty acids consist of a heterogeneous group of fatty acids, containing only carbon-to-carbon single bonds. Saturated fatty acids differ based on the length of the carbon chain, and known as very long-chain, long-chain, medium-chain, and short-chain fatty acids, despite this definition is not standardized. The chain length is increased with the increasing melting points of individual saturated fatty acids (Astrup et al. 2020). Saturated fatty acids of ≥ 10 carbon atoms are solid at room temperature (Ratnayake and Galli 2009). Indeed, the key food contributors of individual saturated fatty acids in the diet also differ by the chain length of saturated fatty acids. For instance, dairy fats are rich in short-chain saturated fatty acids, while long- and medium-chain saturated fatty acids are primarily found in plant oils, dairy fats, and red meat (Ratnayake and Galli 2009; Hu et al. 1999). Intriguingly, the food sources of saturated fatty acids contain various fractions of fatty acids, additionally to other nutrients, which can subsequently affect the biological and physiological effects (Ratnayake and Galli 2009; Mensink et al. 2003). Table 7.1 shows the major dietary sources of SFA.

Saturated fatty acids are also categorized based on the absence or presence of methyl branches on the carbon chain. Branched-chain saturated fatty acids are predominantly found in ruminant-derived foods, beef, and dairy (Ran-Ressler et al. 2014), which exert similar physicochemical properties as unsaturated fatty acids, particularly lower melting points. Intriguingly, branched-chain fatty acids influence the composition of microbiota in the direction of microorganisms that utilize the

Table 7.1 Major dietary sources of SFA

Carbon chain length	Systematic or common name	Abbreviation	Major dietary sources
Short	Butyric	4:0	Dairy foods
Short	Caproic	6:0	Dairy foods
Medium	Caprylic	8:0	Palm kernel and coconut oils, fairy foods
Medium	Capric	10.0	Dairy foods
Medium	Lauric	12:0	Coconut oil and milk
Long	Myristic	14:0	Dairy foods
Long	Pentadecanoic	15:0	Oils, dairy foods, and red meat
Long	Palmitic	16:0	Palm oil, dairy foods, and red meat
Long	Heptadecanoic	17:0	Dairy food, red meat
Long	Stearic	18:0	Chocolate, meat, and dairy foods

fatty acids in cellular membranes (Ran-Ressler et al. 2011), as normal components of the healthy human infant gut (Ran-Ressler et al. 2008).

Circulating saturated fatty acids can also be categorized based on the origin as endogenous or exogenous. In general, circulating amounts of even number-chain saturated fatty acids, for instance stearic, palmitic, and myristic acid are affected by dietary intakes. Yet, they are also endogenously synthesized through de novo lipogenesis, a process in which extra protein and carbohydrates are converted to fatty acids (Wu et al. 2011). In addition, odd number-chain saturated fatty acids including heptadecanoic and pentadecanoic acids are predominantly synthesized by the bacterial flora in the rumen, even though the *in vivo* model suggests that a potential role of endogenous synthesis via elongation of heptanoic and propionic acids (Pfeuffer and Jaudszus 2016). Research evidence from large observational studies demonstrated an inconsistent association between saturated fatty acids with different metabolic, chemical, and physical structures, hence supporting a broad spectrum of different saturated fatty acids on diabetes, insulin resistance, glucose-insulin homeostasis, and blood lipids (Li et al. 2022; Gaeini et al. 2022).

Saturated fats are foods containing predominantly lipids, and solid at temperatures, in which they are customarily consumed and stored. For instance, palm kernel and palm oils, coconut oil, animal fats such as lard and tallow, dairy-derived fats contained in cheese, butterfat, and butter. These fats are solid due to the saturated fatty acids, in which the saturated show specific chemical structural properties of fatty acid, particularly a reduced ability to chemically react to H_2 or I_2. Most of the saturated fatty acids in human diets are lauric, myristic, palmitic, and stearic acids with linear chains of 12, 14, 16, and 18 carbon atoms, respectively (Astrup et al. 2020).

7.3 Polyunsaturated Fatty Acids Oxidation and Lipid Peroxidation

PUFA are critical for the production of a broad spectrum of bioactive compounds in the body, but like several essential minerals and vitamins, may become toxic when consumed in extremely high amounts. PUFAs can be oxidized in a spontaneous chemical oxidation process that does not require enzymes and modulated in cells under normal processes. The spontaneous oxidation is initiated by RNS, ROS, and free radicals, which are constantly generated in biological systems (Tan et al. 2018a; Di Meo 2020). A free radical oxidative process known as lipid peroxidation, requires molecular oxygen, to produce reactive carbonyl species including malondialdehyde, and several other toxic products. The broad spectrum of toxic organic products, RNS, and ROS produced during lipid peroxidation of PUFAs can lead to DNA mutations and subsequently result in cancer (Tan et al. 2018b). Lipid peroxidation can damage cell membranes and cause cell death. Indeed, lipid peroxidation and ROS are implicated in several diseases, aging, and oxidative stress (Tan and Norhaizan 2021).

Lipid peroxidation of PUFAs in lipoproteins, for instance, low-density lipoprotein (LDL), leads to the oxidized LDL being eliminated from the circulation by macrophages lining the arteries, leading to atherosclerosis (Zhong et al. 2019). Undoubtedly, consumption of PUFA is essential as they have well-recognized health benefits, particularly in preventing heart disease (Bender et al. 2014). Nonetheless, it is recommended to have adequate vitamin E to match the high intake of PUFA (Bender et al. 2014). This is due to the lipophilic antioxidant vitamin E which plays a crucial role in protecting PUFA (Niki 2014). Moreover, the previous study has demonstrated that vitamin E requirement is elevated almost proportionally with the unsaturation degree of PUFA (Bender et al. 2014). Mammals preferentially oxidize PUFAs through the β-oxidation pathway in mitochondria to produce ATP, or in peroxisomes to recycle excess PUFAs into MUFAs and SFAs (Lawrence 2021).

7.4   Fatty Acids and Serum Lipids

Inflammatory responses are initiated by a broad spectrum of lipid mediators such as eicosanoids produced from arachidonic acid (AA), the predominant omega-6 long-chain PUFA in membrane phospholipids of immune cells (Dennis and Norris 2015). The biochemical processes that determine the concentration of serum cholesterol are the cholesterol synthesis rate, particularly in the liver, and metabolic intake to produce several steroid products in the body. The gene expression that codes for enzymes for cholesterol and other lipid synthesis is mediated by several gene expressions including sterol regulatory element-binding proteins (SREBPs) (Horton et al. 2002). Multiple phenomena take place to elevate the SREBPs (SREBP2 and SREBP1a) to enhance the gene expression for cholesterol synthesis and uptake from circulating lipoproteins (DeBose-Boyd and Ye 2018). Insulin can also trigger an elevation of nuclear SREBP1 (both SREBP1c and SREBP1a), which will lead to the expression of genes for fatty acids and cholesterol synthesis when carbohydrates are consumed in excess and stored as fat (Lawrence 2021).

7.5   Effects of Fats on Cardiovascular Disease

Evidence from meta-analysis of cohort studies included a study from inception to first July 2018 demonstrated that higher dietary trans fatty acids consumption was linked to increased risk of CVD. Nonetheless, it showed that PUFA, SFA, MUFA, and total fat did not lead to CVD risk. The study further revealed that an increment of 2% energy/day of trans fatty acid consumption elevated 16% of CVD risk (Zhu et al. 2019).

Another meta-analysis and systematic review of prospective cohort studies included 14 studies including 598,435 participants. Intriguingly, the data showed that higher intakes of saturated fatty acids were linked to a reduction in overall stroke risk. However, the data showed that every 10 g/day increase in saturated fatty acid consumption is linked to a 6% relative risk decrease in the rate of stroke (Kang et al. 2020). Ho et al. (2020) found that lower consumption of saturated fat and polyunsaturated fat and higher consumption of monounsaturated fat were associated with a lower risk of mortality, suggesting the diverse and complex associations between macronutrient intake and health outcomes. Similarly, intake of total fat (including MUFA) and total carbohydrates (including sugar) were linearly related to the incidence of CVD (Ho et al. 2020).

A study analyzed of 15 randomized controlled trials involving 56,675 participants revealed that long-term reduction of dietary saturated fat decreased the risk of combined cardiovascular events by 17%, suggesting that a greater reduction in saturated fat consumption resulted in a greater decrease in CVD events risk. The study reviewed demonstrated that decreasing saturated fat consumption for at least 2 years has the potential to reduce combined cardiovascular events (Hooper et al. 2020). Likewise, a meta-analysis and systematic review of prospective cohort studies involving 1,013,273 participants reported that diets high in saturated fat were linked to higher mortality from CVD and all causes. Diets high in saturated fat not only increase CVD but also increase mortality from cancer (Kim et al. 2021). Kim et al. (2021) further showed that a 5% energy increment of intakes in polyunsaturated, monounsaturated, and total fat intakes was negatively linked to all-cause mortality. Diets high in trans fat were linked to higher mortality from CVD and all-cause, while intakes of diets high in monounsaturated fat were related to lower all-cause mortality (Kim et al. 2021). Emerging evidence related high consumption of fat, particularly saturated fat, to the development of CVD risk. Nonetheless, not all evidence showed such a link. Several studies reported by Siri-Tarino et al. (2010), de Souza et al. (2015), Zhu et al. (2019), and Kang et al. (2020) have demonstrated no significant association between mortality or coronary artery disease and saturated fat consumption. Some of these studies also suggested that higher consumption of saturated fat decreased the risk of stroke. Consistent with the studies reported by Siri-Tarino et al. (2010), de Souza et al. (2015), Zhu et al. (2019), Kang et al. (2020), and Korat et al. (2020) also found that biomarkers of very long-chain saturated fatty acids (24:0, 22:0, 20:0) were failed to show any association with nonfatal and fatal coronary heart disease.

Emerging evidence indicates that low-density lipoprotein cholesterol (LDL-C) is a crucial risk factor for atherosclerosis, a main cause of atherosclerotic CVD. Data from systematic review and meta-analysis of cohort studies included 7 cohort studies of ischemic stroke and none of peripheral artery disease, and 13 cohort studies of coronary heart disease (CHD). The study showed that cheese consumption (20 g higher intake/day) was inversely related to CHD and high-fat milk (200 g higher intake/day) was positively linked to CHD, suggesting that a negative link between cheese with CHD risk and a positive link of high-fat milk on CHD risk (Jakobsen et al. 2021).

Very long-chain saturated fatty acids are simple aliphatic (straight) chain fatty acids, which differ from saturated fatty acids such as stearic acid (18:0) and palmitic acid (16:0), based on the dietary sources, biological, and chemistry properties in addition to the length. Canola oil, macadamia nuts, and peanuts are rich in very long-chain saturated fatty acids. A Cardiovascular Health Study (CHS) found that increased plasma phospholipid very long-chain saturated fatty acids are linked to the reduced risk of incident atrial fibrillation (Lemaitre et al. 2018), heart failure (Lemaitre and King 2022), and mortality risk (Lemaitre and King 2022). Atrial fibrillation is a common arrhythmia that influences the synchronicity of the heart rhythm between the heart ventricles and atria. Indeed, the typical quivering of the atrial leads to blood pools that can enhance blood clot formation and elevate the risk of stroke (Lemaitre and King 2022).

7.6   Saturated Fatty Acids and Inflammation

Studies from animal and *in vitro* have shown that SFAs can promote atherosclerosis and trigger inflammation via stimulation of toll-like receptors (Kong et al. 2022). Nonetheless, there is limited evidence on the effects of dietary fatty acids on the inflammatory process in humans. The inflammatory markers including E-selectin and interleukin-6 (IL-6), but not C-reactive protein (CRP), were found to be reduced after consumption of a diet high in oleic acid compared to a diet with 8% of energy as oleic acid substituted with either stearic acid or a combination of palmitic, myristic, and lauric acids (Baer et al. 2004). Nevertheless, no difference in interferon-ɣ, CRP, IL-8, IL-6, IL-1β, tumor necrosis factor-alpha (TNF-α) (Voon et al. 2011) after intakes of diets containing 20% energy with oleic acid-rich olive oil, myristic and lauric acid-rich coconut oil, or palmitic acid-rich palm olein. Likewise, diets containing high PUFAs or SFAs were not linked to the changes in inflammatory markers (Forsythe et al. 2010).

A diet containing high SFA meal has been demonstrated to decrease the ability of high-density lipoprotein (HDL) to suppress vascular cell adhesion molecule-1 and intercellular adhesion molecule-1 expression after 6 h of consumption; whereas HDL collected after intakes of high-PUFA diet suppressed expression to a greater extent than fasting plasma (Nicholls et al. 2006). However, there were no differences were detected in plasma IL-6 and TNF-α after 4-week of dietary intake of a higher-CHO diet supplemented with omega-3 fatty acid, a MUFA-rich Mediterranean diet, or an SFA-rich Western diet (Jiménez-Gómez et al. 2009). Compared to an omega-3 fatty acid-rich diet, a diet high in SFA triggered a greater elevation of TNF-α and IL-6 mRNA in peripheral blood mononuclear cells (Jiménez-Gómez et al. 2009). There are inconsistent research findings, yet most of the studies are limited in meal composition and study population.

Oxidative stress is a crucial player of CVD linked to excessive fat intake. A high-fat diet may act as a stimulus to increase the systemic inflammatory response at the onset of CVD. Taken together, the data demonstrates that high-fat diets activate oxidative stress by increasing inflammatory markers and augmenting the inflammatory response. Substituting total and SFAs with polyunsaturated and monounsaturated fatty acids is linked to a decrease in CVD risk, despite there is heterogeneity in both categories and fatty acids.

References

Ahrens EH Jr, Hirsch J, Insull W Jr et al (1957) Dietary control of serum lipids in relation to atherosclerosis. JAMA J Am Med Assoc 164:1905–1911

Astrup A, Magkos F, Bier DM et al (2020) Saturated fats and health: a reassessment and proposal for food-based recommendations: JACC state-of-the-art review. J Am Coll Cardiol 76:844–857

Baer DJ, Judd JT, Clevidence BA et al (2004) Dietary fatty acids affect plasma markers of inflammation in healthy men fed controlled diets: a randomized crossover study. Am J Clin Nutr 79:969–973

Bender N, Portmann M, Heg Z et al (2014) Fish or n3-PUFA intake and body composition: a systematic review and meta-analysis. Obes Rev 15:657–665

de Souza RJ, Mente A, Maroleanu A et al (2015) Intake of saturated and trans unsaturated fatty acids and risk of all cause mortality, cardiovascular disease, and type 2 diabetes: systematic review and meta-analysis of observational studies. BMJ 351:h3978

DeBose-Boyd RA, Ye J (2018) SREBPs in lipid metabolism, insulin signaling, and beyond. Trends Biochem Sci 43:358–368

Dennis EA, Norris PC (2015) Eicosanoid storm in infection and inflammation. Nat Rev Immunol 15:511–523

Di Meo S, Venditti P (2020) Evolution of the knowledge of free radicals and other oxidants. Oxid Med Cell Longev, volume 2020, Article 9829176, p 32

Fan J, Watanabe T (2022) Atherosclerosis: known and unknown. Pathol Int 72:151–160

FAO (2018) Food-based dietary guidelines: Food and Agriculture Organization of the United Nations. http://www.fao.org/nutrition/education/food-dietary-guidelines/regions/en. Accessed 27 Dec 2018

Forsythe CE, Phinney SD, Feinman RD et al (2010) Limited effect of dietary saturated fat on plasma saturated fat in the context of a low carbohydrate diet. Lipids 45:947–962

Gaeini Z, Bahadoran Z, Mirmiran P (2022) Saturated fatty acid intake and risk of type 2 diabetes: an updated systematic review and dose–response meta-analysis of cohort studies. Adv Nutr 13:2125–2135

Ho FK, Gray SR, Welsh P et al (2020) Associations of fat and carbohydrate intake with cardiovascular disease and mortality: prospective cohort study of UK Biobank participants. BMJ 368:m688

Hooper L, Martin N, Jimoh OF et al (2020) Reduction in saturated fat intake for cardiovascular disease. Cochrane Database Syst Rev 5:CD011737

Horton JD, Goldstein JL, Brown MS (2002) SREBPs: activators of the complete program of cholesterol and fatty acid synthesis in the liver. J Clin Invest 109:1125–1131

Hu FB, Stampfer MJ, Manson JE et al (1999) Dietary saturated fats and their food sources in relation to the risk of coronary heart disease in women. Am J Clin Nutr 70:1001–1008

Ignatowski AC (1908) Influence of animal food on the organism of rabbits. Izvest Imper Voennomed Akad St Petersburg 16:154–173

Jakobsen MU, Trolle E, Outzen M et al (2021) Intake of dairy products and associations with major atherosclerosis cardiovascular diseases: a systematic review and meta-analysis of cohort studies. Sci Rep 11:1303

Jiménez-Gómez Y, López-Miranda J, Blanco-Colio LM et al (2009) Olive oil and walnut break-fasts reduce the postprandial inflammatory response in mononuclear cells compared with a butter breakfast in healthy men. Atherosclerosis 204:e70–e76

Kang Z-Q, Yang Y, Xiao B (2020) Dietary saturated fat intake and risk of stroke: systematic review and dose–response meta-analysis of prospective cohort studies. Nutr Metab Cardiovasc Dis 30:179–189

Kim Y, Je Y, Giovannucci EL (2021) Association between dietary fat intake and mortality from all-causes, cardiovascular disease, and cancer: a systematic review and meta-analysis of prospective cohort studies. Clin Nutr 40:1060–1070

Koneru SC, Sikand G, Agarwala A (2023) Optimizing dietary patterns and lifestyle to reduce atherosclerotic cardiovascular risk among south Asian individuals. Am J Cardiol 203:113–121

Kong P, Cui Z-Y, Huang X-F et al (2022) Inflammation and atherosclerosis: signaling pathways and therapeutic intervention. Signal Transduct Target Ther 7:131

Korat AVA, Qian F, Imamura F et al (2020) Biomarkers of very long-chain saturated fatty acids and incident coronary heart disease: prospective evidence from 15 cohorts in the fatty acids and outcomes research consortium (Abstract P414). Circulation 141:AP414

Lawrence GD (2021) Perspective: the saturated fat–unsaturated oil dilemma: relations of dietary fatty acids and serum cholesterol, atherosclerosis, inflammation, cancer, and all-cause mortality. Adv Nutr 12:647–656

Lemaitre RN, King IB (2022) Very long-chain saturated fatty acids and diabetes and cardiovascular disease. Curr Opin Lipidol 33:76–82

Lemaitre RN, McKnight B, Sotoodehnia N et al (2018) Circulating very long-chain saturated fatty acids and heart failure: the cardiovascular health study. J Am Heart Assoc 7:e010019

Li Z, Lei H, Jiang H et al (2022) Saturated fatty acid biomarkers and risk of cardiometabolic diseases: a meta-analysis of prospective studies. Front Nutr 9:963471

Libby P (2021) The changing landscape of atherosclerosis. Nature 592:524–533

Mensink RP, Zock PL, Kester AD et al (2003) Effects of dietary fatty acids and carbohydrates on the ratio of serum total to HDL cholesterol and on serum lipids and apolipoproteins: a meta-analysis of 60 controlled trials. Am J Clin Nutr 77:1146–1155

Michas G, Micha R, Zampelas A (2014) Dietary fats and cardiovascular disease: putting together the pieces of a complicated puzzle. Atherosclerosis 234:320–328

Mozaffarian D, Micha R, Wallace S (2010) Effects on coronary heart disease of increasing polyunsaturated fat in place of saturated fat: a systematic review and meta-analysis of randomized controlled trials. PLoS Med 7:e1000252

Nations FaAOotU (2010) Summary of conclusions and dietary recommendations on total fat and fatty acids in fats and fatty acids in human nutrition—report of an expert consultation. FAO/WHO, Geneva

Nicholls SJ, Lundman P, Harmer JA et al (2006) Consumption of saturated fat impairs the anti-inflammatory properties of high-density lipoproteins and endothelial function. J Am Coll Cardiol 48:715–720

Niki E (2014) Role of vitamin E as a lipid-soluble peroxyl radical scavenger: *in vitro* and *in vivo* evidence. Free Radic Biol Med 66:3–12

Nowbar AN, Gitto M, Howard JP et al (2019) Mortality from ischemic heart disease: analysis of data from the World Health Organization and coronary artery disease risk factors from NCD risk factor collaboration. Circ Cardiovasc Qual Outcomes 12:e005375

Ordovas JM, Lopez-Miranda J, Mata P et al (1995) Gene-diet interaction in determining plasma lipid response to dietary intervention. Atherosclerosis 118:S11–S27

Pfeuffer M, Jaudszus A (2016) Pentadecanoic and heptadecanoic acids: multifaceted odd-chain fatty acids. Adv Nutr 7:730–734

Ran-Ressler RR, Devapatla S, Lawrence P, Brenna JT (2008) Branched chain fatty acids are constituents of the normal healthy newborn gastrointestinal tract. Pediatr Res 64:605–609

Ran-Ressler RR, Khailova L, Arganbright KM et al (2011) Branched chain fatty acids reduce the incidence of necrotizing enterocolitis and alter gastrointestinal microbial ecology in a neonatal rat model. PLoS One 6:e29032

Ran-Ressler RR, Bae S, Lawrence P et al (2014) Branched-chain fatty acid content of foods and estimated intake in the USA. Br J Nutr 112:565–572

Ratnayake WM, Galli C (2009) Fat and fatty acid terminology, methods of analysis and fat digestion and metabolism: a background review paper. Ann Nutr Metab 55:8–43

SACN (2019) Saturated fats and health. Public Health England, London

Siri-Tarino PW, Sun Q, Hu FB, Krauss RM (2010) Meta-analysis of prospective cohort studies evaluating the association of saturated fat with cardiovascular disease. Am J Clin Nutr 91:535–546

Steinberg D (2004) Thematic review series: the pathogenesis of atherosclerosis. An interpretive history of the cholesterol controversy: part I. J Lipid Res 45:1583–1593

Tan BL, Norhaizan ME (2021) Chapter 3 age-related oxidative stress-induced redox imbalance. The role of antioxidants in longevity and age-related diseases. Springer Nature, Cham, pp 27–38

Tan BL, Norhaizan ME, Liew W-P-P et al (2018a) Antioxidant and oxidative stress: a mutual interplay in age-related diseases. Front Pharmacol 9:1162

Tan BL, Norhaizan ME, Liew W-P-P (2018b) Nutrients and oxidative stress: friend or foe? Oxid Med Cell Longev, volume 2018, Article ID 9719584, p 24

Vazquez-Vidal I, Desmarchelier C, Jones PJH (2019) Nutrigenetics of blood cholesterol concentrations: towards personalized nutrition. Curr Cardiol Rep 21:38

Voon PT, Ng TK, Lee VK et al (2011) Diets high in palmitic acid (16:0), lauric and myristic acids (12:0 + 14:0), or oleic acid (18:1) do not alter postprandial or fasting plasma homocysteine and inflammatory markers in healthy Malaysian adults. Am J Clin Nutr 94:1451–1457

WHO (2018) Draft WHO Guidelines: Saturated fatty acid and trans-fatty intake for adults and children. WHO

World Health Organization (2024) Cardiovascular diseases. https://www.who.int/health-topics/cardiovascular-diseases#tab=tab_1. Accessed 12 Feb 2024

Wu JH, Lemaitre RN, Imamura F et al (2011) Fatty acids in the de novo lipogenesis pathway and risk of coronary heart disease: the cardiovascular health study. Am J Clin Nutr 94:431–438

Zhong S, Li L, Shen X et al (2019) An update on lipid oxidation and inflammation in cardiovascular diseases. Free Radic Biol Med 144:266–278

Zhu Y, Bo Y, Liu Y (2019) Dietary total fat, fatty acids intake, and risk of cardiovascular disease: a dose-response meta-analysis of cohort studies. Lipids Health Dis 18:91

Part II
Pharmacological Insights

Chapter 8
The Role of Diets in Oxidative Stress-Induced Diseases

Oxidative stress is elevated in cancer cells and diabetic patients (Tan and Norhaizan 2021b). A higher concentration of intracellular glucose can produce reactive oxygen species (ROS) via a few mechanisms, and the development and progression of diseases could be prevented by modifying dietary habits. Research evidence has shown that excessive fat intakes and a high animal-based protein and glucose diet can enhance oxidative stress (Tan et al. 2018). For example, excessive omega-6 fatty acids can activate inflammation. In contrast, other dietary choices, such as the Okinawan and Mediterranean diets, common in Japanese and Greek populations, respectively, can decrease inflammation.

8.1 Whole Grains

Whole grains are a primary dietary source of energy, vitamins, lipids, minerals, proteins, complex carbohydrates, dietary fiber, and phytochemicals, offering health benefits beyond basic nutrition (Allai et al. 2022). Their high nutritional value comes from a balanced profile of micro- and macronutrients and amino acids. Approximately 41% of grains are used for human consumption, while up to 35% serve as animal feed (Poutanen et al. 2022). Recognized as a well-balanced dietary option, whole grains possess functional properties that contribute to medical benefits. The growing health-conscious population is increasingly consuming whole grains due to their health-promoting compounds. Emerging research indicates an inverse relationship between whole grain consumption and the risk of metabolic syndromes and diseases (Hu et al. 2023). Thus, the intake of whole grain cereal foods is associated with significant health benefits at the population level, leading to their inclusion in official dietary guidelines in several countries (Miller 2020).

© The Author(s), under exclusive license to Springer Nature Switzerland AG 2024   71
B. L. Tan, M. E. Norhaizan, *Nutrients and Oxidative Stress: Biochemistry Aspects and Pharmacological Insights*, SpringerBriefs in Food, Health, and Nutrition, https://doi.org/10.1007/978-3-031-75319-0_8

Maize, wheat, rice, oats, sorghum, and barley are important cereal crops world-wide. Cereal grains contribute approximately 50% of dietary energy worldwide, and the contribution is relatively higher in developing countries (World Health Organization 2003). The fiber found in whole grains plays a crucial role in the immune system. Fiber influences the microbiota in the gut and thereby affects the immune function. The consumption of whole grains, for instance, sorghum appears to be beneficial to gut microbiota, and indices linked to hypertension, obesity, cancer, inflammation, and oxidative stress (Tan and Norhaizan 2021a, b, c, d). Whole grains are rich in bioactive constituents and protect against oxidative stress, which can lead to inflammation. Phytochemicals found in wheat sprouts may benefit a certain group of the population due to their ability to improve glucose metabolism and combat oxidative stress linked to obesity.

Evidence from meta-analysis has shown that high consumption of whole grains is linked to a decrease in total cancer risk (Aune et al. 2016). In support of this, a Scandinavian HELGA cohort study has demonstrated that whole grain consumption was inversely linked to colorectal cancer incidence (Kyrø et al. 2013). The large NIH-AARP Diet and Health Study involving 478,994 adults from 50 to 71 years of age has demonstrated that intake of whole grains was negatively linked to colorectal cancer incidence (Hullings et al. 2020). Notably, the fiber from grains was related to the reduced incidence of colorectal cancer, especially rectal and distal colon (Hullings et al. 2020). In a study focused on liver cancer outcomes, Liu et al. (2021b) found a relatively low risk of liver cancer and mortality in chronic liver disease for those with a greater intake of whole grains. The anticancer ability of whole grain is mediated through several modes of action such as antioxidants and inducing apoptosis and cell cycle arrest. The intrinsic components such as fermentable carbohydrates, oligosaccharides, resistant starch, and dietary fiber are believed to be protective via the generation of short-chain fatty acids and increasing fecal bulk (Abdullah et al. 2021). Some research evidence has also reached a similar finding, in which brewers' rice, a rice by-product in the rice industry, exerts a unique complex of bioactive constituents to combat colon carcinogenesis (Tan et al. 2015a, b). Anti-inflammatory activity of brewers' rice protects against free radical damage and oxidative stress by enhanced antioxidant enzymes including SOD, MDA, and NO. They also suppressed DNA damage caused by ROS by upregulating the *Nrf2* signaling pathway. Several studies reported by Tan and Norhaizan (2017) and Esa et al. (2013b) further demonstrated that rice by-products have an antiproliferative activity toward cancer. Interestingly, feeding rats with brewers' rice not only decreased the number of aberrant crypt foci (ACF) (Tan et al. 2016); the relative fractions of bioactive constituents in brewers' rice have also been shown to alleviate kidney and liver damage in azoxymethane-induced oxidative stress (Tan et al. 2015c), suggesting that bioactive compounds found in whole grains may attenuate oxidative stress. Table 8.1 summarizes the effect of whole grain intake on metabolic ailments.

Furthermore, germinated brown rice has also been widely studied. Germinated brown rice contains a significant nutritional component. Germinated brown rice has high amounts of vitamins, minerals, and fiber, it is also rich in a wide range of

Table 8.1   The effect of whole grains consumption on human health

Metabolic ailments	Studies (Cell lines/ Animal/Human)	Food sources	Findings	References
Cardiovascular disease	Data from a meta-analysis included 13 animal experiments and 8 human intervention studies	Quinoa	Improved lipid profiles (LDL-cholesterol, total cholesterol, and triglycerides concentrations) in humans	Li et al. (2024)
Cardiovascular disease	37 healthy overweight men (35–70 years, body mass index >25 kg/m^2) completed a 4-week cross-over intervention, separated by a 4-week washout period	Quinoa-enriched bread (containing 20 g of quinoa flour per day)	Does not affect cardiovascular disease risk markers	Li et al. (2018)
Colorectal cancer	Large NIH-AARP diet and health study involving 478,994 adults from 50 to 71 years of age	Whole grain	Inversely associated with colorectal cancer incidence	Hullings et al. (2020)
Liver cancer	National Institutes of Health–American Association of Retired Persons Diet and Health Study	Whole grain	Reduced risk of liver cancer and chronic liver disease mortality	Liu et al. (2021a), b)

LDL low-density lipoprotein

phytochemicals and has drawn attention in the prevention of CVD risk. These bioactive constituents were shown to have antioxidant activities that are suggested to attenuate CVD risk through mediating oxidative stress and hepatic cholesterol metabolism (Esa et al. 2013a; Imam et al. 2014). Another whole grain, quinoa is rich in starchy carbohydrates, gluten-free protein, unsaturated fatty acids, minerals, and dietary fiber (Kahlon et al. 2016). The intakes of quinoa have a beneficial impact on lipid metabolism, insulin sensitivity, and glucose homeostasis. Data from a meta-analysis included 13 animal experiments and 8 human intervention studies demonstrated that quinoa consumption improved lipid profiles including LDL-cholesterol, total cholesterol, and triglycerides concentrations in humans (Li et al. 2024). Li et al. (2024) further demonstrated that quinoa consumption significantly reduced the glucose concentrations. This finding suggests the cardioprotective potential of quinoa intake. Accordingly, natural compounds found in whole grains, for instance, polyphenolic compounds have the potential to inhibit proinflammatory immune signaling and thereby suppress cancer development and improve lipid metabolism.

Gut microbiota plays a vital role in chronic disease, in which the composition is affected by age, genetics, and diet. A close relationship between food intake and microbiota composition exists in long-term dietary habits (Wu et al. 2011). In particular, a high intake of whole grain is linked to a greater microbial variety. It has been shown that high adherence to the Mediterranean diet, a typical eating pattern characterized by a high intake of legumes, vegetables, fruits, and cereals, was linked to the increased anti-inflammatory compounds, for instance, short-chain fatty acids, in fecal samples and decreased atherogenic compounds like trimethylamine N-oxide in urine samples (De Filippis et al. 2016).

Intriguingly, the nutritional values of fiber, for example, β-glucans and arabinoxylans are also present in whole grains. Previous studies have demonstrated a positive association between rye and wheat arabinoxylans and water-soluble maize on caecal fermentation, the production of short-chain fatty acids, and the decrease in serum cholesterol (Ye et al. 2022). Dietary fibers in whole grains also play a crucial role in improving immune function via short-chain fatty acid production, suggesting that increasing the consumption of fermentable dietary fiber may be crucial in decreasing inflammation (Venter et al. 2022). Short-chain fatty acids may boost macrophages, T helper cells, cytotoxic activity, and neutrophils in natural killer cells. Moreover, the fermentation of dietary fiber in the colon and alteration in gut microbiota are linked to impaired gastrointestinal tolerance. The main fermentation pathway generates pyruvate from hexoses in undigested carbohydrates (Slavin 2013). Colonic bacteria utilize a variety of carbohydrates to hydrolyze enzymes and generate hydrogen, short-chain fatty acids (mainly propionate, butyrate, and acetate), methane, lactate, and carbon dioxide. Subsequently, these components stimulate fermentation, increase fecal and bacteria mass, and thereby result in a stool bulking effect (Slavin 2013). Collectively, the data suggests that the protective effect of whole grains on oxidative stress may be partially modulated through additive/synergistic effects of the bioactive constituents present in the whole grains.

8.2   Nuts

Data from epidemiological studies demonstrated that a high frequency of nut intakes was associated with a decreased risk of cardiovascular disease (CVD) (Grosso et al. 2015), nut was brought from obscurity to prominence as a vitally important health food. Since the first epidemiological study in the last decades, scientific evidence on the health effects of nuts has not only centered on the area of coronary heart disease and its risk factors but has also extended to other diseases. Furthermore, evidence from clinical trials revealed that high nut consumption attenuates insulin resistance or endothelial dysfunction and decreases inflammation and oxidative stress (López-Uriarte et al. 2009; Kendall et al. 2010). Consistent study reported by Kris-Etherton (2014), who found a hypocholesterolemic potential of regular intakes of nuts, which partly describes how walnuts decrease the CVD risk.

Despite nuts being energy-dense and high-fat foods, many studies have reported that nuts are rich in bioactive compounds (Ros et al. 2010), that are believed to exert anticarcinogenic and anti-inflammatory properties such as folic acids and some phytochemicals (Bao et al. 2013; Blomhoff et al. 2006). Intriguingly, research evidence suggests that a protective role of nuts in endometrial and colorectal cancer prevention is possible (Nagel et al. 2012; Lux et al. 2012; Yeh et al. 2006).

Data from a meta-analysis included observational studies from inception to March 2020 demonstrated that consumption of total nuts was negatively linked to cancer risk (Naghshi et al. 2021). Such a negative relationship was also found in tree nut consumption. In a further study focused on the dose-response outcomes, an elevation of 5 g/day of total nut intake was linked to 25%, 6%, and 3% lower risk of colon, pancreatic, and overall cancers, respectively. In terms of cancer mortality, higher consumption of peanuts, tree nuts, and total nuts reduced the risk by 8%, 18%, and 13%, respectively. Intriguingly, an elevation of 5 g/day of total nut consumption was associated with a 4% decreased risk of cancer mortality, suggesting a protective association between tree nut or total nut intake on cancer risk and mortality (Naghshi et al. 2021). Despite studies that have shown an inverse association between nuts intake and cancer, not all evidence showed such an association. Fang et al. (2021) did not identify an association between frequent nut consumption and total cancer risk and common individual cancers. Fang et al. (2021) evaluated the associations between total and specific types of nuts intake such as walnut, tree nut, peanut, and tree nuts other than walnut, and total cancer and common cancers risk including aggressive prostate, bladder, breast, colorectal, and lung cancer in 3 large prospective cohorts, and found that nut intake was not associated with the risk of total cancer and common individual cancers.

The unsaturated fatty acids present in nuts contribute to the prevention of CVD and diabetes risk. Conversely, nuts are complex food matrices that are also a source of bioactive compounds including phenolic compounds and tocopherols. In particular, compared to those who never consume nuts or other nuts intake, individuals who consume walnuts have a better CVD risk profile (Yi et al. 2022). Furthermore, individuals with walnut intake had lower fasting blood glucose compared to those with never consumed nuts (Yi et al. 2022). Substantial evidence shows that polyunsaturated fatty acids (PUFAs) and monounsaturated fatty acids (MUFAs) have a greater thermogenic effect (Casas-Agustench et al. 2009) and are more readily oxidized (Piers et al. 2002) than do saturated fatty acids, which may contribute to less fat accumulation. Because nuts contain a unique nonfat and fat composition, they are more likely to modulate inflammation and oxidative stress. It has been shown that inflammation and oxidative stress are mediators in the pathophysiology of numerous chronic diseases (Tan and Norhaizan 2021a, b, c, d). Evidence from randomized clinical trials and cohort studies demonstrate that peanuts and tree nuts have the potential to decrease inflammation and oxidative stress (Rajaram et al. 2023). Furthermore, consumption of tree nuts was found to decrease the risk of cardiovascular outcomes (Martini et al. 2021), mediate vascular tone (Stanisic et al. 2021), modulate energy metabolism (Franco Estrada et al. 2021), and reduce triglycerides, ApoB, LDL cholesterol, and total cholesterol (Del Gobbo et al. 2015). A meta-analysis of randomized clinical trials further revealed that Brazil nut intake improved selenium levels and glutathione peroxidase (GPx) activity, suggesting that Brazil nuts possess antioxidant effects (Godos et al. 2022). The favorable effect could be due to the unique complex of bioactive constituents such as vitamin E,

PUFAs, MUFAs, minerals, phytosterols, polyphenols, and fiber. Selenium is a crucial micronutrient that serves as a component for numerous selenoproteins in redox reactions and antioxidants. Indeed, selenium is essential for the mediation of GPx, which is an antioxidant enzyme that catalyzes lipid hydroperoxide and hydrogen peroxide via glutathione metabolism (Battin and Brumaghim 2009).

In addition, nuts are a highly satiating food due to the abundance of protein, unsaturated fatty acids, and fiber. Subsequently, hunger is decreased and food intake is curtailed after consumption of nuts. The physical structure of nuts may also result in the satiety effect because they must be masticated to small enough before swallowing. Mastication activates mechanical, nutrient, and sensory signaling systems that may modify appetitive sensations (Mattes and Dreher 2010). Evidence from population-based studies demonstrated an inverse association between the consumption of nuts and CRP (Sweazea et al. 2014). IL-6 plasma levels were decreased after intake of a Mediterranean diet with nuts compared to a control diet (Estruch et al. 2006; Colpo et al. 2014). Several studies reported by Zhao et al. (2004) and (2007) assessed walnuts rich in PUFAs such as alpha-linolenic acid (ALA), to inflammatory markers and proinflammatory cytokine generation by blood mononuclear cells. The study found that the CRP levels were decreased by 75% in subjects with an ALA diet compared to the average American diet (Zhao et al. 2004) (Table 8.2). By contrast, CRP levels in subjects consuming the linoleic acid (LA) diet were reduced by 45% (Zhao et al. 2004). In a further study focused on inflammation outcomes, Zhao et al. (2007) found that participants who consumed an ALA-enriched diet decreased inflammatory markers for instance, TNF-α, IL-6, and IL-1β generated by cultured mononuclear cells (Table 8.2).

Based on the data of marine-derived omega-3 PUFA, ALA would be expected to have anti-inflammatory properties. This was described in a clinical study with a relatively small observed effect (Rangel-Huerta et al. 2012). Nonetheless, an *in vitro* study showed that THP-1 cells supplemented with docosahexaenoic acid (DHA), LA, palmitic acid, and ALA in the presence of lipopolysaccharide (Zhao et al. 2005) significantly decreased IL-1β, TNF-α, and IL-6 levels after treatment with ALA, DHA, and LA compared to palmitic acid, suggesting that ALA present in walnuts exerts an anti-inflammatory response. Interestingly, cellular adhesion molecules are biochemical markers of endothelial dysfunction concomitantly with inflammation. A study by Zhao et al. (2007) further compared a diet high in LA, a diet high in ALA, and an American diet, respectively in hypercholesterolemic subjects. The study found that subjects who consumed 15 g of walnut oil and 37 g of walnuts/day for 6 weeks demonstrated a decrease in cellular adhesion molecule soluble intercellular adhesion molecule (sICAM) 1, CRP, and E-selectin. Notably, some evidence has emerged to suggest that CVD risk factors are involved in the mediation of LDL cholesterol and negatively influence endothelial function (Cortés et al. 2006; Lind et al. 2011). Importantly, the acute intakes of walnut oils are favorably affected and demonstrate a better endothelial function (Berryman et al. 2013). Moreover, walnut oil and walnuts may affect inflammation, partly through the increase of cholesterol efflux, which is a reverse cholesterol transport that is important for the removal of cholesterol from peripheral tissues, which implies a cardiovascular effect

Table 8.2 The effect of nuts consumption on human health

Metabolic ailments	Studies (Cell lines/Animal/Human)	Food sources	Findings	References
Cardiovascular disease	Hypercholesterolemic men and women	Walnuts rich in PUFAs such as ALA	CRP levels were decreased by 75% in subjects with an ALA diet compared to the average American diet	Zhao et al. (2004)
Cardiovascular disease	Hypercholesterolemic subjects	ALA-enriched diet	Decreased several inflammatory markers including IL-1β, IL-6, and TNF-α generated by cultured mononuclear cells	Zhao et al. (2007)
Cardiovascular disease	Hypercholesterolemic subjects	15 g of walnut oil and 37 g of walnuts/day for 6 weeks	Decreased in cellular adhesion molecule sICAM 1, CRP, and E-selectin	Zhao et al. (2007)
Cancer	The meta-analysis included observational studies from inception to March 2020	Total nuts	Inversely associated with the risk of cancer	Naghshi et al. (2021)
Cancer	The meta-analysis included observational studies from inception to March 2020	Peanuts or tree nuts, or total nuts	Higher consumption of peanuts, tree nuts, and total nuts reduced the cancer mortality risk by 8%, 18%, and 13%, respectively	Naghshi et al. (2021)
Cancers (aggressive prostate, bladder, breast, colorectal, and lung cancer)	3 large prospective cohorts	Walnut, tree nut, peanut, and tree nut other than walnut	Not associated with the risk of total cancer and common individual cancers	Fang et al. (2021)
Cardiovascular disease	3092 young adults enrolled in the Coronary Artery Risk Development in Young Adults (CARDIA) study	Walnut	Better cardiovascular disease risk profile	Yi et al. (2022)

(continued)

Table 8.2 (continued)

Metabolic ailments	Studies (Cell lines/ Animal/Human)	Food sources	Findings	References
Diabetes	3092 young adults enrolled in the Coronary Artery Risk Development in Young Adults (CARDIA) study	Walnut	Had lower fasting blood glucose compared to those with never consumed nuts	Yi et al. (2022)
Coronary artery disease	25 coronary artery disease patients	One unit of Brazil nut (5 g/day for 3 months)	Did not mitigate inflammation and oxidative stress	de França Cardozo et al. (2021)

ALA alpha-linolenic acid, *CRP* C-reactive protein, *IL-1β* interleukin-1beta, *IL-6* interleukin-6, *PUFAs* polyunsaturated fatty acids, *sICAM 1* soluble intercellular adhesion molecule 1, *TNF-α* tumor necrosis factor-α.

(Kris-Etherton 2014). Collectively, nuts seem a good dietary choice for the prevention of metabolic ailments and obesity as well as providing nutrients. Nevertheless, the phytochemicals that are responsible for the effects mentioned above are worth further investigation.

8.3   Fruits and Vegetables

Fruits and vegetables are rich in vitamins, minerals, and dietary fiber. High consumption of fruits and vegetables is inversely linked to the incidence and mortality of obesity-associated diseases including type 2 diabetes, cancer, and CVD (Partula et al. 2020; Liu et al. 2021a, b; Wang et al. 2021). This favorable effect could be attributed to the antioxidant vitamins, for instance, vitamin E, β-carotene, and vitamin C. Importantly, more than 85% of the total antioxidants in fruits and vegetables are hydrophilic antioxidants. Vitamins C and E and β-carotene are crucial for the proper modulation of physiological function. Vitamin E is well-recognized for maintaining the oxidant-antioxidant balance. Vitamin C can improve the antioxidant protection. Beta-carotene is often present in bright-colored fruits and vegetables. It exerts an ability to reduce LDL-cholesterol oxidation and maintain the immune system via the mediation of antioxidant enzymes (Tan and Norhaizan 2021a, b, c, d). In addition to the vitamin antioxidants mentioned above, several dietary compounds including flavonoids may protect against oxidative stress. Flavonoids are plant polyphenolic compounds ubiquitous in vegetables and fruits. Flavonoids possess many biological activities including antioxidant activity, antitumor effects, antimicrobial action, and anti-inflammatory activity, and they inhibit platelet aggregation (Tan et al. 2018).

The animal model study has shown that a diet enriched with β-carotene from fruits significantly decreased the acetyl-CoA carboxylase, fatty acid synthase, and fat synthesis-related gene expression (Jin et al. 2017). Data from population-based studies have corroborated some of the preclinical findings obtained from an *in vivo* study. Findings from a population-based study revealed that high consumption of vegetables and fruits significantly reduced body weight, energy consumption, sagittal abdominal diameter, and waist circumference in obese and overweight women and men (Järvi et al. 2016). Table 8.3 shows the effects of consumption of fruits and vegetables on chronic diseases.

Data from epidemiological studies have demonstrated that fruit and vegetable consumption triggers protective cardiometabolic effects. A study reported by Wood et al. (2017) found that encapsulated vegetable and fruit-concentrated juice reduced plasma TNF-α, total cholesterol, systolic blood pressure, and LDL-cholesterol, and increased total lean mass. Such improvements have been accredited to the alteration of transcriptional activity of NF-κB and AMP-activated protein kinase (AMPK) (Wood et al. 2017). Blood lipids, body composition, and systemic inflammation were improved in obese participants after fruit and vegetable intake and thereby providing a useful approach for decreasing obesity-induced metabolic ailments. Moreover, vegetables and fruits can also assist in the restoration of morphology and function of the heart and vessels after injury and prevent CVDs. Vegetables and fruits are believed to protect against CVD by attenuating ischemia/reperfusion injury, suppressing thrombosis, inhibiting platelet function, modulating lipid metabolism, decreasing oxidative stress, alleviating inflammation, mediating blood pressure, and protecting vascular endothelial function (Zhao et al. 2017a; Farràs et al. 2016).

Besides its effects on CVD and obesity, a beneficial effect of vegetable and fruit intake in humans has also been demonstrated on the incidence of type 2 diabetes. Findings from a meta-analysis included a study from 1966 to 2014 has found that high fruit consumption, especially berries, and cruciferous, yellow, green leafy vegetables or their fibers, is inversely associated with type 2 diabetes (Wang et al. 2016). For instance, lactucaxanthin (Lxn), a carotenoid in lettuce (*Lactuca sativa*), inhibits α-glucosidase and α-amylase activity in both diabetic rats and *in vitro* model (Gopal et al. 2017). These findings indicate the role of unique complexes of bioactive compounds in vegetables and fruits.

In addition to the effects observed on CVD, obesity, and diabetes, fruits and vegetables have the potential to protect against cancers, demonstrating the numerous functional potentials of vegetables and fruits. Data from epidemiological studies have demonstrated fruit and vegetable intake is negatively linked to cancer risks including breast, colon, and prostate cancers. This inhibitory effect was primarily found in cruciferous and green-yellow vegetables (Aune et al. 2017) through the mediation of transcription factors involved in glucose metabolism and proliferation and the induction of some antioxidant genes (Huang et al. 2016). Several studies have also reached a similar finding, in which fruits and vegetables have the potential to protect against cancers. A systematic review and meta-analysis including 34 case-control studies and 15 cohort studies demonstrated that consumption of fruits and vegetables was associated with a 29% lower risk of breast cancer, respectively (Shin et al. 2023). Intriguingly, dietary fiber in vegetables and fruits undergo fermentation by gut microbiota, which may result in short-chain fatty acid production.

Table 8.3 The effect of fruit and vegetable intakes on human health

Metabolic ailments	Studies (Cell lines/Animal/ Human)	Food sources	Findings	References
Breast cancer	A systematic review and meta-analysis including 34 case-control studies and 15 cohort studies	Fruits and vegetables	Associated with 29% lower risk of breast cancer, respectively	Shin et al. (2023)
Obesity	Beef cattle	A diet enriched with β-carotene from fruits	Significantly decreased the acetyl-CoA carboxylase, fatty acid synthase, and fat synthesis-related gene expression	Jin et al. (2017)
Obesity	Obese and overweight women and men	Vegetables and fruits	Significantly reduced body weight, energy consumption, sagittal abdominal diameter, and waist circumference	Järvi et al. (2016)
Obesity-induced systemic inflammation	Obese participants	Encapsulated vegetable and fruit-concentrated juice	Reduced plasma TNF-α, total cholesterol, systolic blood pressure, and LDL-cholesterol and increased total lean mass	Wood et al. (2017)
Type 2 diabetes	The meta-analysis included a study from 1966 to 2014	Fruit consumption, especially berries, and cruciferous, yellow, green leafy vegetables or their fibers	Inversely associated with type 2 diabetes	Wang et al. (2016)
Type 2 diabetes	Diabetic rats	Lactucaxanthin (Lxn), a carotenoid in lettuce (*Lactuca sativa*)	Inhibits α-glucosidase and α-amylase activity	Gopal et al. (2017)
Cancer	A systematic review and dose-response meta-analysis of prospective studies	Fruits and vegetables	Negatively linked to cancer risks including breast, colon, and prostate cancers	Aune et al. (2017)

Short-chain fatty acids including butyrate (Han et al. 2017), acetate (Schug et al. 2016), and propionic acids (Yang et al. 2017) may exert protective effects against cancers. It would be possible that certain types of fruits and vegetables confer protection against oxidative stress. Since several bioactive constituents modulate the same transcription factor and signaling pathways targeted by drugs, diets high in fruits and vegetables in combination with medical therapies are being regarded as a novel treatment approach (Ristow 2014). Taken together, bioactive compounds in vegetables and fruits might be a promising approach for the attenuation of numerous chronic diseases (Alissa and Ferns 2017).

8.4 Fish and Meat

8.4.1 Fish

Fish is a crucial source of omega-3 fatty acids, dietary protein, and minerals. Compared to those with underweight or normal weight, individuals who consume fish daily were negatively linked to obesity (Nakamura et al. 2016). The consumption of fish has been associated with a decreased metabolic syndrome risk (Karimi et al. 2020), and the fish composition usually includes representative amounts of PUFA, for instance, n-3 fatty acids, in which the chemical structure makes them susceptible to peroxidation and are present abundantly in fatty fish. Hence, the body is prone to oxidative stress and thereby stimulates the lipid peroxidation process. Undoubtedly, PUFA consumption is vitally important as they have well-established health benefits, particularly in preventing heart disease. Nonetheless, it is recommended to consume adequate vitamin E to match the elevation of PUFA consumption (Raederstorff et al. 2015). This could be due to the lipophilic antioxidant vitamin E plays a crucial role in protecting PUFA. Furthermore, a study reported by Raederstorff et al. (2015) demonstrated that vitamin E requirement is elevated almost proportionally with the degree of unsaturation of the PUFA.

Emerging evidence indicates that the intake of lean fish possesses beneficial effects on glucose homeostasis, insulin sensitivity, and lipid metabolism (Aadland et al. 2015; Rylander et al. 2014). Notably, data from population-based study has shown that consumption of lean fish for 4 weeks reduced the very low-density lipoprotein (VLDL) levels, decreased the ratio of total to high-density lipoprotein (HDL) cholesterol in serum, and decreased postprandial and fasting triacylglycerol (TAG) compared to those individuals with a nonseafood diet, suggesting the cardioprotective potential of lean-seafood consumption (Aadland et al. 2015). In support of this, Schmedes et al. (2016) further demonstrated that lean seafood intakes decreased the urinary excretion of metabolites involved in energy metabolism and mitochondrial lipid in healthy subjects, possibly facilitating higher lipid catabolism. Importantly, lean fish contains a relatively low amount of marine n-3 fatty acids. In this regard, the beneficial effects of fish are not solely ascribed to the composition of lipids.

In addition, dietary protein has been suggested as the most effective food macronutrient to provide a satiating effect. Hence, protein-rich foods are involved in promoting body weight loss, mediation of food intake, and maintaining body weight thereafter. The release of glucagon-like peptide-1 (GLP-1) activated by a high-protein meal is triggered by carbohydrates. Moreover, the release of peptide YY (PYY) and cholecystokinin (CCK) is also stimulated by a high-protein meal (Morell and Fiszman 2017).

Fish not only exerts macronutrients but also contains a variety of antioxidant sources due to its composition and provides a relatively low amount of saturated fat compared to other food items. Taurine, an amino acid that is abundantly present in fish, is a crucial antioxidant source. Taurine can effectively combat metabolic syndrome by regulating the kallikrein-kinin and renin-angiotensin-aldosterone systems to reduce blood pressure, regulating glucose metabolism, lowering cholesterol (particularly decreasing LDL + VLDL cholesterol and increasing HDL cholesterol), and decreasing triglycerides to prevent diet-induced hypercholesterolemia (Chen et al. 2016).

Intriguingly, the generation of fish protein peptides (hydrolysates) maximizes the usage of fish protein because peptides exert health-promoting potential (Halim et al. 2016). The procedures, for instance, thermal hydrolysis, autolysis, and enzymatic hydrolysis have been developed to produce fish hydrolysates. The beneficial roles of fish hydrolysates such as neuroprotective, antitumor-, antimicrobial-, cardioprotective- (antiatherosclerotic, antihypertensive, and anticoagulant), immunomodulatory-, antioxidative-, analgesic-, antiviral-, and appetite-suppressing activities have drawn tremendous interest from the pharmaceutical industry, which attempts to design the prevention and treatment of several diseases (Pangestuti and Kim 2017).

Besides fish protein peptides and fish, both *in vivo* and *in vitro* studies showed that neovastat (AE-941), a liquid extract derived from the cartilage of sharks, possesses anti-inflammatory, antiangiogenic, and antitumor properties (Yadav et al. 2014). Such favorable effects are modulated through the inhibition of matrix metalloproteinases (MMP)-9, MMP-2, and MMP-12 and the stimulation of tissue plasminogen activator enzymatic activities (Yadav et al. 2014).

In addition to the effects mentioned above, fish has the potential to protect against cancers. Data from a systematic review and meta-analysis of 29 studies involving 1,475,125 participants and 18,836 cases of bladder cancer revealed a higher consumption of fish was inversely associated with the risk of bladder cancer (Yu et al. 2023) (Table 8.4). Furthermore, a similar dietary intake was found to decrease the risk of hepatocellular carcinoma (Yu et al. 2022). Taken together, it remains unknown whether PUFA or its antioxidant is responsible for the beneficial effects. Further study is warranted to conclusively elucidate the question behind the anti-inflammatory effects of fish.

Table 8.4 The effect of fish and meat on human health

Metabolic ailments	Studies (Cell lines/ Animal/Human)	Food sources	Findings	References
Multiple cancer	72 meta-analyses	Red meat	100 g/day increment increased by 11–51% multiple cancer risk	Huang et al. (2021)
Multiple cancer	72 meta-analyses	Processed meat	50 g/day increment increased by 8–72% multiple cancer risk	Huang et al. (2021)
Prostate cancer	Systematic review and meta-analysis (25 prospective studies (1,900,910 participants with 35,326 incident cases of prostate cancer))	Total meat and processed meat	May link to a higher risk of prostate cancer	Nouri-Majd et al. (2022)
Breast cancer	Systematic review and meta-analysis from inception to December 2022 involving 34 case-control studies and 15 cohort studies	Meat	Not significantly associated with breast cancer risk	Shin et al. (2023)
Colorectal adenoma and lung cancer	Meta-analyses of prospective cohort studies	Total meat	Excessive intake of total meat increases the risk of colorectal adenoma and lung cancer	Grosso et al. (2022)
Colorectal adenoma, ovarian, prostate, renal, and stomach cancers	Meta-analyses of prospective cohort studies	Red meat	Increased risk of cancers	Grosso et al. (2022)
Colon and bladder cancers	Meta-analyses of prospective cohort studies	Processed meat	Increased risk of cancers	Grosso et al. (2022)
Bladder cancer	A systematic review and meta-analysis included 29 studies involving 1,475,125 participants and 18,836 cases of bladder cancer	Fish	Inversely associated with the risk of bladder cancer	Ye et al. (2022)

(continued)

Table 8.4 (continued)

Metabolic ailments	Studies (Cell lines/ Animal/Human)	Food sources	Findings	References
Bladder cancer	A systematic review and meta-analysis included 29 studies involving 1,475,125 participants and 18,836 cases of bladder cancer	White meat	No association	Ye et al. (2022)
Bladder cancer	A systematic review and meta-analysis included 29 studies involving 1,475,125 participants and 18,836 cases of bladder cancer	Total meat	Increased risk of cancer	Ye et al. (2022)
Bladder cancer	A systematic review and meta-analysis included 29 studies involving 1,475,125 participants and 18,836 cases of bladder cancer	Processed meat or red meat	High intakes may increase the risk of bladder cancer	Ye et al. (2022)
Hepatocellular carcinoma	Meta-analysis (17 studies involving 2,915,680 participants and 4953 cases of hepatocellular carcinoma)	Red meat and total meat	Not associated with the risk of hepatocellular carcinoma	Yu et al. (2022)
Hepatocellular carcinoma	Meta-analysis (17 studies involving 2,915,680 participants and 4953 cases of hepatocellular carcinoma)	Processed meat	Higher intakes may increase the risk of hepatocellular carcinoma	Yu et al. (2022)
Hepatocellular carcinoma	Meta-analysis (17 studies involving 2,915,680 participants and 4953 cases of hepatocellular carcinoma)	White meat and fish	Inversely associated with cancer risk	Yu et al. (2022)

(continued)

Table 8.4 (continued)

Metabolic ailments	Studies (Cell lines/Animal/Human)	Food sources	Findings	References
Cardiovascular disease	Randomized controlled trial with a crossover design (healthy subjects)	Lean fish (4 weeks)	Reduced VLDL levels, decreased the ratio of total to HDL cholesterol in serum, and decreased postprandial and fasting TAG	Aadland et al. (2015)
Coronary heart disease and stroke	Meta-analyses of prospective cohort studies	Total meat	High intakes of total meat increase the risk of coronary heart disease and stroke	Grosso et al. (2022)
Coronary heart disease and stroke	Meta-analyses of prospective cohort studies	Red meat	Increased risk of coronary heart disease and stroke	Grosso et al. (2022)
Coronary heart disease	Prospective cohort study	Total meat	Increased 53% of 10-year coronary heart disease risk	Jeong et al. (2023)
Coronary heart disease	Prospective cohort study	Red meat	Increased 55% of 10-year coronary heart disease risk	Jeong et al. (2023)
Coronary heart disease	Prospective cohort study	Processed meat or poultry	No association on 10-year coronary heart disease risk	Jeong et al. (2023)
Stroke	Prospective cohort studies	Unprocessed red meat and processed meat	Associated with the incidence of stroke	de Medeiros et al. (2022)
Cardiovascular disease	Prospective cohort studies	Unprocessed red meat and processed meat	No positive association in cardiovascular disease mortality	de Medeiros et al. (2022)
Type 2 diabetes	Human hepatocytes	Heterocyclic amines	Significantly increases in gluconeogenic genes	Walls et al. (2021)

HDL high-density lipoprotein, *TAG* triacylglycerol, *VLDL* very low-density lipoprotein

8.4.2   Meat

Meat is a crucial component of the human diet. Meat contains many minerals, vitamins, and essential amino acids, thereby making it an excellent source of protein. Although there is a minor difference in the animal's age, diet, and species, saturated fatty acids (SFAs) usually comprise nearly half the fat in meat. Importantly, meat contributes to almost half of the maximal recommended intake of SFAs (Wyness et al. 2011; Council 2014). Therefore, the high composition of SFA has become a spotlight in recent decades. The previous study has shown that the world per capita intake of red meat has increased to 36.4 kg/year (1999) from 24.2 kg/year (1964) (Bruinsma 2003). The per capita intake of meat is projected to increase by up to 45.3% (Bruinsma 2003). The rapid rise in meat consumption has had a negative impact on public health and thereby leads to an increase in colorectal cancer, cardiovascular disease (CVD), diabetes, and obesity (Richi et al. 2015).

Despite meat products being a predominant source of high biological value protein; yet, meat products and meat are perishable food that require additives to prevent rapid deterioration and to ensure the absence of pathogenic bacteria and foodborne microorganisms. Lipid oxidation is one of the primary contributors to quality deterioration in meat products and meat (Tatiyaborworntham et al. 2022). This reaction results in a reduction of sensory quality and nutritional value of meat products. The changes during oxidation could affect the safety of the product or influence consumer acceptance (appearance of rancid flavor and odor, and texture and color alteration) (Sottero et al. 2019). In this regard, intake of processed meat (meats transformed via smoking, fermentation, curing, salting, or other processes to improve preservation or enhance flavor) and red meats (meats of mammalian origin such as lamb, pork, and beef) has been increasing rapidly globally (Godfray et al. 2018; GBD 2017 Diet Collaborators 2019; Willett et al. 2019). These trends may contribute to environmental and health consequences (Qian et al. 2020). Data from several large observational studies have shown a positive association between high consumption of processed and red meat and the risk of type 2 diabetes, all-cause mortality, cancer, and CVD (Shi et al. 2023; Zhong et al. 2020). However, heterogeneity and risk-of-bias analyses found that the observed association between processed and red meat and an increased risk of diseases seen in meta-analyses of observational studies may be attributed to confounders (Zhao et al. 2017a, b; Yip et al. 2018; Händel et al. 2019, 2020; Han et al. 2019). Such finding indicates the extrapolation from observational studies should be performed with caution when exploring the health effects of meat among populations with major differences in food culture. Some research emerged to suggest that certain nutrients in meat may not contribute an effect per se, but the overall consumption of the matrix from the meals and the diet are more likely to mediate or lead to adverse outcomes (Geiker et al. 2021). Indeed, several factors such as cooking practices (Góngora et al. (2019), calcium (López et al. 2014), and fiber (Ward et al. 2016) are more likely to be strong effect modulators when evaluating meat and disease, and the inclusion factors and study quality linked to the different food cultures surrounding meat consumption could play a crucial role (Han et al. 2019). In the context of the environment, livestock production, especially ruminant animals, causes the vast majority of greenhouse gas emissions attributable to the agricultural sector, which accounts for 22% of global total emissions, and results in environmental degradation through desertification, deforestation, and fertilizer run-off (McMichael et al. 2007).

Considerable evidence indicates that the majority of existing dietary guidelines such as the *Dietary Guidelines for Americans 2015–2020* (U.S. Department of Health and Human Services and U.S. Department of Agriculture 2015), recommend a dietary pattern high in minimally processed plant foods and relatively low in processed and red meats. A consensus report from the American Diabetes Association recommends several dietary patterns for managing and preventing type 2 diabetes, most of which emphasize no or modest consumption of processed or red meats (Evert et al. 2019). These include the vegetarian/plant-based regimens (Kahleova et al. 2017; Willett et al. 2019; Qian et al. 2019), the traditional Mediterranean-style diet (Estruch et al. 2018), and the Dietary Approaches to Stop Hypertension (DASH) (Sacks et al. 2001). Furthermore, The American College of Cardiology/American Heart Association Guideline on the Primary Prevention of Cardiovascular Disease also recommends consuming a diet low in processed and red meats (Arnett et al. 2019). Notably, the International Agency for Research on Cancer (IARC) categorized processed meat as a Group 1 carcinogen for human colorectal cancer, and red meat was categorized as probably carcinogenic to humans (Group 2A) based on the data from a comprehensive review of epidemiologic evidence, combined with "strong mechanistic evidence supporting a carcinogenic effect" (Bouvard et al. 2015). From the study reviewed, the IARC has recommended decreasing processed and red meat consumption for cancer prevention. A collection of meta-analyses and systematic reviews along with the dietary guidelines by the "Nutritional Recommendations (NutriRECS) consortium," has challenged these recommendations (Johnston et al. 2019; Han et al. 2019; Vernooij et al. 2019; Zeraatkar et al. 2019; Valli et al. 2019). The study found that most people are generally unwilling to shift their current meat intake habits. Further, the data also indicates that individuals should be advised to continue their current intake habits of meat due to the "low certainty" of the finding, the weak associations, and the difficulty of modifying meat eaters' preferences and habits.

The epidemiological study indicates that high intakes of well-done meat could increase the risk of cancer because cooking protein-rich foods such as fish and meat at high temperatures can result in carcinogenic compounds like polycyclic aromatic hydrocarbon (PAHs) and heterocyclic amines (HCAs) (Zheng and Lee 2009). The systematic review and meta-analysis of prospective studies included a study from inception to December 2020 involving 35,326 incident cases of prostate cancer and 1,900,910 participants revealed that increased consumption of processed meat and total meat may be associated with a higher risk of prostate cancer (Nouri-Majd et al. 2022). The study further demonstrated that an increment in consumption of 50 g per day of processed meat may be linked to a 4% greater risk of total prostate cancer (Nouri-Majd et al. 2022). A study by Grosso et al. (2022) demonstrated that excessive consumption of total meat increases the risk of colorectal adenoma and lung cancer. High intakes of red meat also increase the risk of stomach, renal, prostate, and ovarian cancers, and colorectal adenoma (Table 8.4). Furthermore, meta-analyses of prospective cohort studies found that excessive consumption of processed meat is positively associated with the risk of bladder and colon cancers (Grosso et al. 2022). These findings suggested that excessive meat intake may be detrimental to health, particularly in cancers. In another meta-analysis involving 1,475,125 participants and 18,836 cases of bladder cancer, Ye et al. (2022) found an increased risk for bladder cancer for those with total meat intake. The study further demonstrated that a higher consumption of processed meat or red meat may increase the risk of bladder cancer (Yu et al. 2023) (Table 8.4). However, Yu et al. (2022) did not identify an association between white meat and the risk of bladder cancer. A similar dietary intake of white meat was also found to be negatively associated with the risk of hepatocellular carcinoma (Yu et al. 2022). The data from systematic review and meta-analysis included a study from inception to December 2022 involving 34 case-control studies and 15 cohort studies further demonstrating that meat consumptions were not significantly associated with breast cancer risk (Shin et al. 2023). Yu et al. (2022) explored the relationship between meat intake and hepatocellular carcinoma risk in the meta-analysis of observational studies. The data showed that consumption of red meat and total meat was not linked to the risk of hepatocellular carcinoma. Nonetheless, a higher processed meat consumption may increase the hepatocellular carcinoma risk.

In addition to the effects observed on cancers, excessive intake of total meat also increased the risk of stroke and coronary heart disease. The study showed that high red meat consumption is positively associated with the risk of stroke and coronary heart disease (Grosso et al. 2022). Further, the data from the Korean Genome and Epidemiology Study (KoGES) Health Examinees (HEXA) study involving 13,293 Korean male adults demonstrated that individuals with the highest total meat consumption increased by 53% of 10-year coronary heart disease risk compared to the lowest intake of total meat (Jeong et al. 2023). Compared to those with the lowest intake of red meat, subjects with the highest consumption of red meat increased 55% of 10-year coronary heart disease risk (Jeong et al. 2023). Nonetheless, Jeong et al. (2023) did not identify an association between processed meat or poultry intake and 10-year coronary heart disease risk. These findings suggest that consumption of red meat and total meat was linked to a higher risk of coronary heart disease in Korean male adults. In another systematic review and meta-analysis of prospective cohort studies, de Medeiros et al. (2022) found that unprocessed red meat and processed meat intakes are linked to the incidence of stroke (Table 8.4). However, de Medeiros et al. (2022) did not identify a positive association between unprocessed red meat and processed meat intake to cardiovascular disease mortality.

Diabetes mellitus is suffered by the elderly and can cause a severe complication including diabetic peripheral neuropathy. A study reported by Walls et al. (2023) showed that high intake of heterocyclic amine (HCA) increased the prevalence of insulin resistance, a hallmark of metabolic syndrome and type 2 diabetes mellitus. HCA mutagens are produced in meats cooked at high temperatures (Khan et al. 2022). HCA was further divided into two classes, namely amino amidazo azoarenes and amino carbolines (Jägerstad et al. 1983). Many factors influence the formation of HCAs during cooking such as pre-treatment procedures, precursors in meat, fat content, type of cooking oil used, method of cooking, cooking temperature, and cooking time. Walls et al. (2021) evaluated HCA exposure to insulin sensitivity by inducing primary human hepatocytes and hepatocellular carcinoma (HepG2) cells with 2-amino-3,4-dimethylimidazo[4,5-f]quinoline (MeIQ). The study showed that the HepG2 cells exposed to MeIQ reduced insulin-induced p-AKT levels in low glucose conditions, suggesting that the cells become insulin resistance in the presence of MeIQ. It has been demonstrated that MeIQ significantly upregulated the transcriptional factors involved in gluconeogenesis such as *PCK1* and *G6PC* in

HepG2 cells. Compared to vehicle-treated cells, primary human hepatocytes exposed to MeIQ significantly upregulated gluconeogenic genes (Walls et al. 2021). This finding indicates that MeIQ potentially triggers glucose production in hepatocytes and impairs insulin signaling. Taken together, meat is a good source of vitamins, minerals, proteins, as well as other crucial components. The currently available evidence is inconclusive and does not support the association between meat intake and increased risk of diseases. Furthermore, the lack of interventional studies and the potential confounding factors may influence the effect of meat consumption on health. Indeed, processed meat should be eaten moderately. Excessive intake of processed red meat (smoked and cured) may carry the risk of developing several diseases or intensifying existing ones.

8.5 Legumes

Legumes are a main component of the Mediterranean diet. Legumes are rich in protein and fiber, which can facilitate decreasing the glycemic response and lowering energy density. They also contain minerals including calcium, potassium, iron, and B vitamins. Indeed, most of the nutritional value in legumes is contributed by relative fractions of fibers, protein, and phytochemicals including lectins, saponins, isoflavones, phenolic compounds, oligosaccharides, and phytoestrogens. Consumption of legumes has been reported to have beneficial effects in the prevention of several related disorders and obesity due to their high nutritional values (Moreno-Valdespino et al. 2020).

The previous study has shown that adults who consume legumes significantly reduce waist circumference and body mass index compared to those who never or rarely consume legumes. Children who consume legumes show smaller waist circumferences compared to those who never consume legumes (Garcia-Bailo et al. 2017). A study reported by Shinohara et al. (2016) further showed that ethanol extracts of chickpeas improved gene expression related to fatty acid metabolism in adipocytes and total lipid indices. It has been demonstrated that enzymes involved in lipogenesis, for instance, acetyl-CoA carboxylase (ACC), AMPK, and liver kinase B1 (LKB1) were inactivated by phosphorylation. Moreover, lipolysis was affected by the ethanol extracts of chickpeas by increasing the uncoupling protein 2 (UCP2) and carnitine palmitoyltransferase 1 (CPT1), which is a protein or an enzyme important for fatty acid oxidation (Shinohara et al. 2016), suggesting that Desi-type chickpeas may effective for treating diabetes.

Starch composition and digestibility affect glycemic response. Legumes are high in amylose starch. However, the digestion of high amylose starch is significantly decreased compared to high amylopectin starch (Miao et al. 2013). A study reported by Yang et al. (2015) showed a more sustainable plasma glucose level after consuming a high-amylose meal compared to a high-amylopectin meal. Importantly, legumes have a high protein level; therefore, the interaction of protein-starch may further hamper digestibility (Bhattarai et al. 2017). Furthermore, high dietary fiber

Table 8.5 The effect of legume intake on human health

Metabolic ailments	Studies (Cell lines/Animal/Human)	Food sources	Findings	References
Breast cancer	Systematic review and meta-analysis included a study from inception to December 2022 involving 34 case-control studies and 15 cohort studies	Soy isoflavone and soy protein	Significantly decreased the risk of breast cancer	Shin et al. (2023)
Breast cancer	Systematic review and meta-analysis included a study from inception to December 2022 involving 34 case-control studies and 15 cohort studies	Soy food	No significant	Shin et al. (2023)
CVD	Systematic review and meta-analysis	Legume	6% lowered risk of CVD compared to the lowest legume intake	Marventano et al. (2017)

CVD cardiovascular disease

significantly decreased the rate and extent of legume starch digestibility. A high consumption of fiber may improve insulin resistance, promote satiety, and reduce the glycemic response (Grundy et al. 2016). Data from epidemiological studies demonstrated that consumption of legumes is inversely linked to fasting glucose levels (Dhillon et al. 2016). Table 8.5 summarizes the effect of legume consumption on human health.

In addition to the effects observed above, a protective effect of legumes has also been documented on the cancers. For instance, soy food protects against estrogen receptor-negative breast cancer (Guo et al. 2016). Women with high consumption of soy show an upregulation of tumor suppressor genes (IGF1R and miR-29a-3p) and a downregulation of oncogenes (FGFR4 and KRAS) (Guo et al. 2016). In support of this, green pea- (*Pisum sativum*) extracted lectin exerts antiproliferative activity toward liver cancer cell lines (El-Aassar et al. 2014). Data from systematic review and meta-analysis included a study from inception to December 2022 involving 34 case-control studies and 15 cohort studies demonstrating that high consumption of soy isoflavone and soy protein significantly decreased the risk of breast cancer (Shin et al. 2023). However, intakes of soy food were not significantly associated with breast cancer risk (Shin et al. 2023).

Although the limited available data to draw a firm conclusion, several studies suggest that legumes may be potentially beneficial to certain population segments. Taken together, further investigations are warranted to elucidate the role of legumes in human health, yet their use in a balanced diet should be considered in the absence of clear contraindications.

References

Aadland EK, Lavigne C, Graff IE et al (2015) Lean-seafood intake reduces cardiovascular lipid risk factors in healthy subjects: results from a randomized controlled trial with a crossover design. Am J Clin Nutr 102:582–592

Abdullah MMH, Hughes J, Grafenauer S (2021) Whole grain intakes are associated with healthcare cost savings following reductions in risk of colorectal cancer and total cancer mortality in Australia: a cost-of-illness model. Nutrients 13:2982

Alissa EM, Ferns GA (2017) Dietary fruits and vegetables and cardiovascular diseases risk. Crit Rev Food Sci Nutr 57:1950–1962

Allai FM, Azad ZRAA, Gul K et al (2022) Whole grains: a review on the amino acid profile, mineral content, physicochemical, bioactive composition and health benefits. Int J Food Sci Technol 57:1849–1865

Arnett DK, Blumenthal RS, Albert MA et al (2019) ACC/AHA guideline on the primary prevention of cardiovascular disease: a report of the American College of Cardiology/American Heart Association task force on clinical practice guidelines. Circulation 140:e596–e646

Aune D, Keum N, Giovannucci E et al (2016) Whole grain consumption and risk of cardiovascular disease, cancer, and all cause and cause specific mortality: systematic review and dose-response meta-analysis of prospective studies. BMJ 353:i2716

Aune D, Giovannucci E, Boffetta P et al (2017) Fruit and vegetable intake and the risk of cardiovascular disease, total cancer and all-cause mortality—a systematic review and dose response meta-analysis of prospective studies. Int J Epidemiol 46:1029–1056

Bao Y, Han J, Hu FB et al (2013) Association of nut consumption with total and cause-specific mortality. N Engl J Med 369:2001–2011

Battin EE, Brumaghim JL (2009) Antioxidant activity of sulfur and selenium: a review of reactive oxygen species scavenging, glutathione peroxidase, and metal-binding antioxidant mechanisms. Cell Biochem Biophys 55:1–23

Berryman CE, Grieger JA, West SG et al (2013) Acute consumption of walnuts and walnut components differentially affect postprandial lipemia, endothelial function, oxidative stress, and cholesterol efflux in human with mild hypercholesterolemia. J Nutr 143:788–794

Bhattarai RR, Dhital S, Wu P et al (2017) Digestion of isolated legume cells in a stomach-duodenum model: three mechanisms limit starch and protein hydrolysis. Food Funct 8:2573–2582

Blomhoff R, Carlsen MH, Andersen LF et al (2006) Health benefits of nuts: potential role of antioxidants. Br J Nutr 96:S52–S60

Bouvard V, Loomis D, Guyton KZ et al (2015) International Agency for Research on Cancer monograph working group. Carcinogenicity of consumption of red and processed meat. Lancet Oncol 16:1599–1600

Bruinsma J (2003) World agriculture: towards 2015/2030. An FAO Perspective. Earthscan Publications Ltd., London

Casas-Agustench P, López-Uriarte P, Bullo M et al (2009) Acute effects of three high-fat meals with different fat saturations on energy expenditure, substrate oxidation and satiety. Clin Nutr 28:39–45

Chen W, Guo J, Zhang Y et al (2016) The beneficial effects of taurine in preventing metabolic syndrome. Food Funct 7:1849–1863

Colpo E, Vilanova CDDA, Reetz LGB et al (2014) Brazilian nut consumption by healthy volunteers improves inflammatory parameters. Nutrition 30:459–465

Cortés B, Núñez I, Cofán M et al (2006) Acute effects of high-fat meals enriched with walnuts or olive oil on postprandial endothelial function. J Am Coll Cardiol 48:1666–1671

Council N (2014) In: Nordic Co-Operation (ed) Nordic nutrition recommendations 2012: integrating nutrition and physical activity, Copenhagen

De Filippis F, Pellegrini N, Vannini L et al (2016) High-level adherence to a Mediterranean diet beneficially impacts the gut microbiota and associated metabolome. Gut 65:1812–1821 de França Cardozo LFM, Mafra D, da Silva ACT et al (2021) Effects of a Brazil nut-enriched diet on oxidative stress and inflammation markers in coronary artery disease patients: a small and preliminary randomised clinical trial. Nutr Bull 46:139–148

de Medeiros GCBS, Mesquita GXB, Lima SCVC et al (2022) Associations of the consumption of unprocessed red meat and processed meat with the incidence of cardiovascular disease and mortality, and the dose-response relationship: a systematic review and meta-analysis of cohort studies. Crit Rev Food Sci Nutr 63(27):8443–8456

Del Gobbo LC, Falk MC, Feldman R et al (2015) Effects of tree nuts on blood lipids, apolipoproteins, and blood pressure: systematic review, meta-analysis, and dose-response of 61 controlled intervention trials. Am J Clin Nutr 102:1347–1356

Dhillon PK, Bowen L, Kinra S et al (2016) Legume consumption and its association with fasting glucose, insulin resistance and type 2 diabetes in the Indian migration study. Public Health Nutr 19:3017–3026

El-Aassar M, Hafez EE, El-Deeb NM et al (2014) Microencapsulation of lectin anti-cancer agent and controlled release by alginate beads, biosafety approach. Int J Biol Macromol 69:88–94

Esa NM, Abdul Kadir K-K, Amom Z et al (2013a) Antioxidant activity of white rice, brown rice and germinated brown rice (*in vivo* and *in vitro*) and the effects on lipid peroxidation and liver enzymes in hyperlipidaemic rabbits. Food Chem 141:1306–1312

Esa NM, Ling TB, Peng LS (2013b) By-products of rice processing: an overview of health benefits and applications. J Rice Res 1:107

Estruch R, Martínez-González MA, Corella D et al (2006) Effects of a Mediterranean-style diet on cardiovascular risk factors: a randomized trial. Ann Intern Med 145:1–11

Estruch R, Ros E, Salas-Salvadó J et al (2018) PREDIMED study investigators. Primary prevention of cardiovascular disease with a Mediterranean diet supplemented with extra-virgin olive oil or nuts. N Engl J Med 378:e34

Evert AB, Dennison M, Gardner CD et al (2019) Nutrition therapy for adults with diabetes or prediabetes: a consensus report. Diabetes Care 42:731–754

Fang Z, Wu Y, Li Y et al (2021) Association of nut consumption with risk of total cancer and 5 specific cancers: evidence from 3 large prospective cohort studies. Am J Clin Nutr 114:1925–1935

Farràs M, Basterra-Gortari FJ, Diez-Espino J et al (2016) Association between dietary fibre intake and fruit, vegetable or whole-grain consumption and the risk of CVD: results from the PREvención con DIeta MEDiterránea (PREDIMED) trial. Br J Nutr 116:534–546

Franco Estrada YM, Caldas APS, da Silva A et al (2021) Effects of acute and chronic nuts consumption on energy metabolism: a systematic review of randomised clinical trials. Int J Food Sci Nutr 73(3):296–306

Garcia-Bailo B, Jain N, Keeler C et al (2017) Legume consumption, diet quality and body weight: results from NHANES 2009–2012 and the food patterns equivalent database 2009–2012. FASEB J 31:615–648

GBD 2017 Diet Collaborators (2019) Health effects of dietary risks in 195 countries, 1990–2017: a systematic analysis for the global burden of disease study 2017. Lancet 393:1958–1972

Geiker NRW, Bertram HC, Mejborn H et al (2021) Meat and human health—current knowledge and research gaps. Food Secur 10:1556

Godfray HCJ, Aveyard P, Garnett T et al (2018) Meat consumption, health, and the environment. Science 361:eaam5324

Godos J, Giampieri F, Micek A et al (2022) Effect of Brazil nuts on selenium status, blood lipids, and biomarkers of oxidative stress and inflammation: a systematic review and meta-analysis of randomized clinical trials. Antioxidants 11:403

Góngora VM, Matthes KL, Castaño PR et al (2019) Dietary heterocyclic amine intake and colorectal adenoma risk: a systematic review and meta-analysis. Cancer Epidemiol Biomarkers Prev 28:99–109

Gopal SS, Lakshmi MJ, Sharavana G et al (2017) Lactucaxanthin—a potential anti-diabetic carotenoid from lettuce (Lactuca sativa) inhibits α-amylase and α-glucosidase activity in vitro and in diabetic rats. Food Funct 8:1124–1131

Grosso G, Yang J, Marventano S et al (2015) Nut consumption on all-cause, cardiovascular, and cancer mortality risk: a systematic review and meta-analysis of epidemiologic studies. Am J Clin Nutr 101:783–793

Grosso G, La Vignera S, Condorelli RA et al (2022) Total, red and processed meat consumption and human health: an umbrella review of observational studies. Int J Food Sci Nutr 73:726–737

Grundy MM-L, Edwards CH, Mackie AR et al (2016) Re-evaluation of the mechanisms of dietary fibre and implications for macronutrient bioaccessibility, digestion and postprandial metabolism. Br J Nutr 116:816–833

Guo X, Cai Q, Bao P et al (2016) Long-term soy consumption and tumor tissue microRNA and gene expression in triple-negative breast cancer. Cancer 122:2544–2551

Halim NRA, Yusof HM, Sarbon NM (2016) Functional and bioactive properties of fish protein hydolysates and peptides: a comprehensive review. Trends Food Sci Technol 51:24–33

Han A, MacDonald A, Ahmed B et al (2017) Butyrate regulates its own metabolic fate as an HDAC inhibitor in colorectal cancer cells. FASEB J 31:300–302

Han MA, Zeraatkar D, Guyatt GH et al (2019) Reduction of red and processed meat intake and cancer mortality and incidence: a systematic review and meta-analysis of cohort studies. Ann Intern Med 171:711–720

Händel MN, Cardoso I, Rasmussen KM et al (2019) Processed meat intake and chronic disease morbidity and mortality: an overview of systematic reviews and meta-analyses. PLoS One 14:e0223883

Händel MN, Rohde JF, Jacobsen R et al (2020) Processed meat intake and incidence of colorectal cancer: a systematic review and meta-analysis of prospective observational studies. Eur J Clin Nutr 74:1132–1148

Hu H, Zhao Y, Feng Y et al (2023) Consumption of whole grains and refined grains and associated risk of cardiovascular disease events and all-cause mortality: a systematic review and dose-response meta-analysis of prospective cohort studies. Am J Clin Nutr 117:149–159

Huang Y, Su Z, Wu T et al (2016) Mechanisms of prostate carcinogenesis and its prevention by a γ-tocopherol-rich mixture of tocopherols in TRAMP mice. J Chin Pharm Sci 25:170–177

Huang Y, Cao D, Chen Z et al (2021) Red and processed meat consumption and cancer outcomes: umbrella review. Food Chem 356:129697

Hullings AG, Sinha R, Liao LM et al (2020) Whole grain and dietary fiber intake and risk of colorectal cancer in the NIH-AARP diet and health study cohort. Am J Clin Nutr 112:603–612

Imam MU, Ishaka A, Ooi D-J et al (2014) Germinated brown rice regulates hepatic cholesterol metabolism and cardiovascular disease risk in hypercholesterolaemic rats. J Funct Foods 8:193–203

Jägerstad M, Reuterswärd AL, Olsson R et al (1983) Creatin(in)e and Maillard reaction products as precursors of mutagenic compounds: effects of various amino acids. Food Chem 12:255–264

Järvi A, Karlström B, Vessby B et al (2016) Increased intake of fruits and vegetables in overweight subjects: effects on body weight, body composition, metabolic risk factors and dietary intake. Br J Nutr 115:1760–1768

Jeong J, Lim K, Shin S (2023) The association between meat intake and the risk of coronary heart disease in Korean men using the Framingham risk score: a prospective cohort study. Nutr Metab Cardiovasc Dis 33:1158–1166

Jin Q, Zhao HB, Liu XM et al (2017) Effect of β-carotene supplementation on the expression of lipid metabolism-related genes and the deposition of back fat in beef cattle. Anim Prod Sci 57:513–519

Johnston BC, Zeraatkar D, Han MA et al (2019) Unprocessed red meat and processed meat consumption: dietary guideline recommendations from the nutritional recommendations (NutriRECS) consortium. Ann Intern Med 171:756–764

Kahleova H, Levin S, Barnard N (2017) Cardio-metabolic benefits of plant-based diets. Nutrients 9:E848

Kahlon TS, Avena-Bustillos RJ, Chiu M-CM (2016) Sensory evaluation of gluten-free quinoa whole grain snacks. Heliyon 2:e00213

Karimi G, Heidari Z, Firouzi S et al (2020) A systematic review and meta-analysis of the associa-
    tion between fish consumption and risk of metabolic syndrome. Nutr Metab Cardiovasc Dis
    30:717–729
Kendall CW, Josse AR, Esfahani A et al (2010) Nuts, metabolic syndrome and diabetes. Br J Nutr
    104:465–473
Khan IA, Khan A, Zou Y et al (2022) Heterocyclic amines in cooked meat products, shortcom-
    ings during evaluation, factors influencing formation, risk assessment and mitigation strategies.
    Meat Sci 184:108693
Kris-Etherton PM (2014) Walnuts decrease risk of cardiovascular disease: a summary of efficacy
    and biologic mechanisms. J Nutr 144:547S–554S
Kyrø C, Skeie G, Loft S et al (2013) Intake of whole grains from different cereal and food sources
    and incidence of colorectal cancer in the Scandinavian HELGA cohort. Cancer Causes Control
    24:1363–1374
Li L, Lietz G, Bal W et al (2018) Effects of quinoa (*Chenopodium quinoa* Willd.) consumption on
    markers of CVD risk. Nutrients 10:777
Li L, Lietz G, Seal CJ (2024) Effects of quinoa intake on markers of cardiovascular risk: a system-
    atic literature review and meta-analysis. Food Rev Int 40:1–19
Lind L, Berglund L, Larsson A et al (2011) Endothelial function in resistance and conduit arteries
    and 5-year risk of cardiovascular disease. Circulation 123:1545–1551
Liu W, Hu B, Dehghan M et al (2021a) Fruit, vegetable, and legume intake and the risk of all-
    cause, cardiovascular, and cancer mortality: a prospective study. Clin Nutr 40:4316–4323
Liu X, Yang W, Petrick JL et al (2021b) Higher intake of whole grains and dietary fiber are associ-
    ated with lower risk of liver cancer and chronic liver disease mortality. Nat Commun 12:6388
López PJT, Albero JS, Rodríguez-Montes JA (2014) Primary and secondary prevention of colorec-
    tal cancer. Clin Med Insights Gastroenterol 7:33–46
López-Uriarte P, Bulló M, Casas-Agustench P et al (2009) Nuts and oxidation: a systematic review.
    Nutr Rev 67:497–508
Lux S, Scharlau D, Schlörmann W et al (2012) *In vitro* fermented nuts exhibit chemopreventive
    effects in HT29 colon cancer cells. Br J Nutr 108:1177–1186
Martini D, Godos J, Marventano S et al (2021) Nut and legume consumption and human health: an
    umbrella review of observational studies. Int J Food Sci Nutr 72:871–878
Marventano S, Pulido MI, Sánchez-González C et al (2017) Legume consumption and CVD risk:
    a systematic review and meta-analysis. Public Health Nutr 20:245–254
Mattes RD, Dreher ML (2010) Nuts and healthy body weight maintenance mechanisms. Asia Pac
    J Clin Nutr 19:137–141
McMichael AJ, Powles JW, Butler CD et al (2007) Food, livestock production, energy, climate
    change, and health. Lancet 370:1253–1263
Miao M, Jiang B, Cui SW et al (2013) Slowly digestible starch-a review. Crit Rev Food Sci Nutr
    55:1642–1657
Miller KB (2020) Review of whole grain and dietary fiber recommendations and intake levels in
    different countries. Nutr Rev 78:29–36
Morell P, Fiszman S (2017) Revisiting the role of protein-induced satiation and satiety. Food
    Hydrocoll 68:199–210
Moreno-Valdespino CA, Luna-Vital D, Camacho-Ruiz RM et al (2020) Bioactive proteins and
    phytochemicals from legumes: mechanisms of action preventing obesity and type-2 diabetes.
    Food Res Int 130:108905
Nagel JM, Brinkoetter M, Magkos F et al (2012) Dietary walnuts inhibit colorectal cancer growth
    in mice by suppressing angiogenesis. Nutrition 28:67–75
Naghshi S, Sadeghian M, Nasiri M et al (2021) Peanut butter consumption with cancer incidence
    and mortality: a comprehensive systematic review and dose-response meta-analysis of obser-
    vational studies. Adv Nutr 12:793–808
Nakamura M, Ojima T, Nakade M et al (2016) Poor oral health and diet in relation to weight loss,
    stable underweight, and obesity in community-dwelling older adults: a cross-sectional study
    from the JAGES 2010 project. J Epidemiol 26:322–329

Nouri-Majd S, Salari-Moghaddam A, Aminianfar A et al (2022) Association between red and processed meat consumption and risk of prostate cancer: a systematic review and meta-analysis. Front Nutr 9:801722

Pangestuti R, Kim S-K (2017) Bioactive peptide of marine origin for the prevention and treatment of noncommunicable diseases. Mar Drugs 15:67

Partula V, Deschasaux M, Druesne-Pecollo N et al (2020) Associations between consumption of dietary fibers and the risk of cardiovascular diseases, cancers, type 2 diabetes, and mortality in the prospective NutriNet-Santé cohort. Am J Clin Nutr 112:195–207

Piers LS, Walker KZ, Stoney RM et al (2002) The influence of the type of dietary fat on postprandial fat oxidation rates: monounsaturated (olive oil) vs saturated fat (cream). Int J Obes Relat Metab Disord 26:814–821

Poutanen KS, Kårlund AO, Gómez-Gallego C et al (2022) Grains—a major source of sustainable protein for health. Nutr Rev 80:1648–1663

Qian F, Liu G, Hu FB et al (2019) Association between plant-based dietary patterns and risk of type 2 diabetes: a systematic review and meta-analysis. JAMA Intern Med 179:1335–1344

Qian F, Riddle MC, Wylie-Rosett J et al (2020) Red and processed meats and health risks: how strong is the evidence? Diabetes Care 43:265–271

Raederstorff D, Wyss A, Calder PC et al (2015) Vitamin E function and requirements in relation to PUFA. Br J Nutr 114:1113–1122

Rajaram S, Damasceno NRT, Braga RAM et al (2023) Effect of nuts on markers of inflammation and oxidative stress: a narrative review. Nutrients 15:1099

Rangel-Huerta O, Aguilera CM, Mesa MD et al (2012) Omega-3 long-chain polyunsaturated fatty acids supplementation on inflammatory biomarkers: a systematic review of randomised clinical trials. Br J Nutr 107:S159–S170

Richi EB, Baumer B, Conrad B et al (2015) Health risks associated with meat consumption: a review of epidemiological studies. Int J Vitam Nutr Res 85:70–78

Ristow M (2014) Unraveling the truth about antioxidants: mitohormesis explains ROS-induced health benefits. Nat Med 20:709–711

Ros E, Tapsell LC, Sabaté J (2010) Nuts and berries for heart health. Curr atheroscler Rep 12:397–406

Rylander C, Sandanger TM, Engeset D et al (2014) Consumption of lean fish reduces the risk of type 2 diabetes mellitus: a prospective population based cohort study of Norwegian women. PLoS One 9, Article e89845:1–10

Sacks FM, Svetkey LP, Vollmer WM et al (2001) DASH-sodium collaborative research group. Effects on blood pressure of reduced dietary sodium and the Dietary Approaches to Stop Hypertension (DASH) diet. N Engl J Med 344:3–10

Schmedes M, Aadland EK, Sundekilde UK et al (2016) Lean-seafood intake decreases urinary markers of mitochondrial lipid and energy metabolism in healthy subjects: metabolomics results from a randomized crossover intervention study. Mol Nutr Food Res 60:1661–1672

Schug ZT, Voorde JV, Gottlieb E (2016) The metabolic fate of acetate in cancer. Nat Rev Cancer 16:708–717

Shi W, Huang X, Schooling CM et al (2023) Red meat consumption, cardiovascular diseases, and diabetes: a systematic review and meta-analysis. Eur Heart J 44:2626–2635

Shin S, Fu J, Shin W-K et al (2023) Association of food groups and dietary pattern with breast cancer risk: a systematic review and meta-analysis. Clin Nutr 42:282–297

Shinohara S, Gu Y, Yang Y et al (2016) Ethanol extracts of chickpeas alter the total lipid content and expression levels of genes related to fatty acid metabolism in mouse 3T3-L1 adipocytes. Int J Mol Med 38:574–584

Slavin J (2013) Fiber and prebiotics: mechanisms and health benefits. Nutrients 5:1417–1435

Sottero B, Leonarduzzi G, Testa G et al (2019) Lipid oxidation derived aldehydes and oxysterols between health and disease. Eur J Lipid Sci Technol 121:1700047

Stanisic J, Ivkovic T, Romic S et al (2021) Beneficial effect of walnuts on vascular tone is associated with Akt signalling, voltage-dependent calcium channel LTCC and ATP-sensitive potassium channel Kv1.2. Int J Food Sci Nutr 72:324–334

Sweazea KL, Johnston CS, Ricklefs KD et al (2014) Almond supplementation in the absence of dietary advice significantly reduces C-reactive protein in subjects with type 2 diabetes. J Funct Foods 10:252–259

Tan BL, Norhaizan ME (2017) Scientific evidence of rice by-products for cancer prevention: chemopreventive properties of waste products from rice milling on carcinogenesis *in vitro* and *in vivo*. BioMed Res Int., Article ID 9017902:18

Tan BL, Norhaizan ME (2021a) Chapter 3 age-related oxidative stress-induced redox imbalance. In: The role of antioxidants in longevity and age-related diseases. Springer Nature, Cham, pp 27–38

Tan BL, Norhaizan ME (2021b) Chapter 5 implications of inflammation in aging and age-related diseases. In: The role of antioxidants in longevity and age-related disease. Springer Nature, Cham, pp 51–80

Tan BL, Norhaizan ME (2021c) Chapter 6 antioxidant and age-related diseases. In: The role of antioxidants in longevity and age-related diseases. Springer, pp 81–156

Tan BL, Norhaizan ME (2021d) Chapter 7 the role of antioxidant on health and age-related diseases in aging. In: The role of antioxidants in longevity and age-related diseases. Springer Nature, Cham, pp 157–276

Tan BL, Norhaizan ME, Huynh K et al (2015a) Brewers' rice modulates oxidative stress in azoxymethane-mediated colon carcinogenesis in rats. World J Gastroenterol 21:8826–8835

Tan BL, Norhaizan ME, Huynh K et al (2015b) Water extract of brewers' rice induces apoptosis in human colorectal cancer cells via activation of caspase-3 and caspase-8 and downregulates the Wnt/β-catenin downstream signaling pathway in brewers' rice-treated rats with azoxymethane-induced colon carcinogenesis. BMC Complement Altern Med 15:205

Tan BL, Norhaizan ME, Hairuszah I et al (2015c) Brewers' rice: a by-product from rice processing provides natural hepatoprotection in azoxymethane-induced oxidative stress in rats. Oxid Med Cell Longev., Article ID 539798:10

Tan BL, Norhaizan ME, Pandurangan AK et al (2016) Brewers' rice attenuated aberrant crypt foci developing in colon of azoxymethane-treated rats. Pak J Pharm Sci 29:205–212

Tan BL, Norhaizan ME, Liew W-P-P et al (2018) Antioxidant and oxidative stress: a mutual interplay in age-related diseases. Front Pharmacol 9:1162

Tatiyaborworntham N, Oz F, Richards MP et al (2022) Paradoxical effects of lipolysis on the lipid oxidation in meat and meat products. Food Chem: X 14:100317

U.S. Department of Health and Human Services and U.S. Department of Agriculture (2015) 2015–2020 Dietary Guidelines for Americans, 8th edn. Available from https://health.gov/dietaryguidelines/2015/guidelines/. Accessed 14 Nov 2019

Valli C, Rabassa M, Johnston BC et al (2019) NutriRECS working group. Health-related values and preferences regarding meat consumption: a mixed-methods systematic review. Ann Intern Med 171:742–755

Venter C, Meyer RW, Greenhawt M et al (2022) Role of dietary fiber in promoting immune health–an EAACI position paper. Eur J Allergy Clin Immunol 77:3185–3198

Vernooij RWM, Zeraatkar D, Han MA et al (2019) Patterns of red and processed meat consumption and risk for cardiometabolic and cancer outcomes: a systematic review and meta-analysis of cohort studies. Ann Intern Med 171:732–741

Walls K, Hong K, Hein D (2021) Changes in insulin signaling and gluconeogenic gene expression in human hepatocytes following exposure to heterocyclic amines. FASEB J 35(S1)

Walls KM, Hong KU, Hein DW (2023) Induction of glucose production by heterocyclic amines is dependent on N-acetyltransferase 2 genetic polymorphism in cryopreserved human hepatocytes. Toxicol Lett 383:192–195

Wang PY, Fang JC, Gao ZH et al (2016) Higher intake of fruits, vegetables or their fiber reduces the risk of type 2 diabetes: a meta-analysis. J Diabetes Investig 7:56–69

Wang DD, Li Y, Bhupathiraju SN et al (2021) Fruit and vegetable intake and mortality: results from 2 prospective cohort studies of US men and women and a meta-analysis of 26 cohort studies. Circulation 143:1642–1654

Ward HA, Norat T, Overvad K et al (2016) Pre-diagnostic meat and fibre intakes in relation to colorectal cancer survival in the European prospective investigation into cancer and nutrition. Br J Nutr 116:316–325

Willett W, Rockström J, Loken B et al (2019) Food in the Anthropocene: the EAT-lancet commission on healthy diets from sustainable food systems. Lancet 393:447–492

Wood LG, Williams EJ, Berthon BS et al (2017) Effects of an encapsulated fruit and vegetable juice concentrate on obesity-induced systemic inflammation. FASEB J 31:161–166

World Health Organization, Food and Agriculture Organization of the United Nations (2003) Diet, nutrition and the prevention of chronic diseases. Report of a joint WHO/FAO expert consultation. WHO technical report series 916. WHO, Geneva. http://www.fao.org/3/ac911e/ac911e00.htm. Accessed 28 Oct 2020

Wu GD, Chen J, Hoffmann C et al (2011) Linking long-term dietary patterns with gut microbial enterotypes. Science 334:105–109

Wyness L, Weichselbaum E, O'Connor A et al (2011) Red meat in the diet: an update. Nutr Bull 36:34–77

Yadav L, Puri N, Rastogi V et al (2014) Matrix metalloproteinases and cancer-roles in threat and therapy. Asian Pac J Cancer Prev 15:1085–1091

Yang C, Chen D, Yu B et al (2015) Effect of dietary amylose/amylopectin ratio on growth performance, carcass traits, and meat quality in finishing pigs. Meat Sci 108:55–60

Yang Y, Nirmagustina DE, Kumrungsee T et al (2017) Feeding of the water extract from Ganoderma lingzhi to rats modulates secondary bile acids, intestinal microflora, mucins, and propionate important to colon cancer. Biosci Biotechnol Biochem 81:1796–1804

Ye S, Shah BR, Li J et al (2022) A critical review on interplay between dietary fibers and gut microbiota. Trends Food Sci Technol 124:237–249

Yeh C-C, You S-L, Chen C-J et al (2006) Peanut consumption and reduced risk of colorectal cancer in women: a prospective study in Taiwan. World J Gastroenterol 12:222–227

Yi S-Y, Steffen LM, Zhou X et al (2022) Association of nut consumption with CVD risk factors in young to middle-aged adults: the coronary artery risk development in young adults (CARDIA) study. Nutr Metab Cardiovasc Dis 32:2321–2329

Yip CSC, Lam W, Fielding R (2018) A summary of meat intakes and health burdens. Eur J Clin Nutr 72:18–29

Yu J, Liu Z, Liang D et al (2022) Meat intake and the risk of hepatocellular carcinoma: a meta-analysis of observational studies. Nutr Cancer 74:3340–3350

Yu J, Li H, Liu Z et al (2023) Meat intake and the risk of bladder cancer: a systematic review and meta-analysis of observational studies. Nutr Cancer 75:825–845

Zeraatkar D, Johnston BC, Bartoszko J et al (2019) Effect of lower versus higher red meat intake on cardiometabolic and cancer outcomes: a systematic review of randomized trials. Ann Intern Med 171:721–731

Zhao G, Etherton TD, Martin KR et al (2004) Dietary α-linolenic acid reduces inflammatory and lipid cardiovascular risk factors in hypercholesterolemic men and women. J Nutr 134:2991–2997

Zhao G, Etherton TD, Martin KR et al (2005) Anti-inflammatory effects of polyunsaturated fatty acids in THP-1 cells. Biochem Biophys Res Commun 336:909–917

Zhao G, Etherton TD, Martin KR et al (2007) Dietary alpha-linolenic acid inhibits proinflammatory cytokine production by peripheral blood mononuclear cells in hypercholesterolemic subjects. Am J Clin Nutr 85:385–391

Zhao C-N, Meng X, Li Y et al (2017a) Fruits for prevention and treatment of cardiovascular diseases. Nutrients 9:598

Zhao Z, Feng Q, Yin Z et al (2017b) Red and processed meat consumption and colorectal cancer risk: a systematic review and meta-analysis. Oncotarget 8:83306–83314

Zheng W, Lee S-A (2009) Well-done meat intake, heterocyclic amine exposure, and cancer risk. Nutr Cancer 61:437–446

Zhong VW, Horn LV, Greenland P et al (2020) Associations of processed meat, unprocessed red meat, poultry, or fish intake with incident cardiovascular disease and all-cause mortality. JAMA Intern Med 180:503–512

Chapter 9
Summary and Future Prospects

Nutrients play a crucial role in mediating oxidative stress levels within the body and subsequently leading to the progression and development of oxidative stress-induced diseases. Oxidative stress is characterized by an imbalance between antioxidant defense mechanisms and reactive oxygen species (ROS), which is implicated in many pathological conditions such as cancer, diabetes mellitus, neurodegenerative disorders, and cardiovascular disease (CVD). Diets rich in antioxidants, for instance, carotenoids, flavonoids, zinc, selenium, vitamin E, and vitamin C, can alleviate oxidative damage and scavenge reactive oxygen species (ROS). In contrast, diets high in unhealthy fats, refined sugars, and processed foods can exacerbate oxidative stress, thereby increasing the risk of chronic diseases (Tan et al. 2018).

The interplay between oxidative stress and nutrients and chronic diseases is multifaceted and involves intricate modes of action. Antioxidants play a crucial role in scavenging reactive oxygen species (ROS), suppressing oxidative damage to cellular components including DNA, proteins, and lipids, and modulating redox-sensitive signaling pathways, thereby possessing protective effects against chronic diseases. Furthermore, certain nutrients exert anti-inflammatory and anticancer properties, further alleviating chronic diseases and oxidative stress (Tan and Norhaizan 2021).

Reactive oxygen species (ROS) are produced as a by-product of several endogenous and exogenous factors, which may trigger oxidative damage to proteins, lipids, and DNA, and subsequently result in cellular dysfunction (Juan et al. 2021). Among all the proinflammatory mediators, cytokines and chemokines are the main contributors to chronic inflammation (Molnar et al. 2021). Oxidative stress is enhanced by several other reactive species, for instance, H_2O_2, $\bullet O_2^-$, and singlet oxygen as well as other non-radicals, which are generated continuously in the body and subsequently modify cellular activity and basic structural components (Tan et al. 2018).

The directions of future studies in this field encompass assessing the specific roles of individual nutrients and the synergistic effects in mediating chronic disease outcomes and oxidative stress. In addition, personalized nutrition strategies based on disease profiles, lifestyle factors, and individual genetic predispositions hold great promise in optimizing dietary interventions for oxidative stress-related diseases. Moreover, exploring novel antioxidant sources from functional foods and natural compounds may unveil alternative approaches for enhancing health outcomes and combating oxidative stress. In this regard, integrating dietary recommendations with lifestyle modifications, for instance, stress management techniques and regular physical activity can also promote longevity and improve the overall resilience against oxidative stress.

The available studies have provided evidence of the identification of known sources of nutritionally mediated oxidative stress as a modulating pathway for obesity and oxidative stress-induced diseases. Oxidative stress has been identified as a key risk factor in the development of several chronic diseases such as cancer, type 2 diabetes, and coronary heart disease, associated with excessive fat intakes and high animal-based protein and carbohydrate diets (Tan et al. 2018). Although discrepant findings support the clinical use of antioxidant agents in preventing the progression and onset of metabolic ailments, for instance, cancer and diabetic complications, most clinical research evidence is limited in their sample size and duration of study. Yet, several preclinical studies in animal experiments and *in vitro* have shown in-depth insight into the mediation of chronic diseases. Taken together, more randomized clinical trials are required to elucidate the overall long-term effects of dietary intervention.

References

Juan CA, de la Lastra JMP, Plou FJ et al (2021) The chemistry of reactive oxygen species (ROS) revisited: outlining their role in biological macromolecules (DNA, lipids and proteins) and induced pathologies. Int J Mol Sci 22:4642

Molnar V, Matišić V, Kodvanj I et al (2021) Cytokines and chemokines involved in osteoarthritis pathogenesis. Int J Mol Sci 22:9208

Tan BL, Norhaizan ME (2021) Chapter 6 antioxidant and age-related diseases. In: The role of antioxidants in longevity and age-related diseases. Springer Nature, Cham, pp 81–156

Tan BL, Norhaizan ME, Liew W-P-P (2018) Nutrients and oxidative stress: friend or foe? Oxid Med Cell Longev, Volume 2018, Article ID 9719584, p 24

Conclusion

This book provides clear evidence that a diet high in fats, animal protein, and carbohydrates leads to the generation of reactive oxygen species (ROS), resulting in oxidative stress. Oxidative stress plays a vitally important role in the development of dementia, metabolic syndromes, cancer, osteoporosis, arthritis, atherosclerosis, diabetes, and vascular diseases. It has been suggested that overproduction of ROS may cause the formation of mutagen compounds and increase oncogene, and subsequently induce inflammation and proatherogenic activity. Inconsistent findings support the beneficial effects of antioxidant agents in delaying and preventing the progression and onset of metabolic ailments, and most clinical studies are limited in the sample size and the duration of the study. Hence, greater adherence to healthy dietary patterns is encouraging and may relate to a lower risk of oxidative stress-induced diseases. The best dietary advice for the management and prevention of metabolic ailments and obesity includes replacing saturated and total fats with monounsaturated fatty acids (MUFAs), substituting refined carbohydrates with whole grains, consuming a moderate amount of calories, and increasing vegetables and fruits with an ultimate goal of maintaining an ideal body weight. In this regard, several anti-inflammatory dietary sources, for instance, legumes, fruits and vegetables, whole grains, dairy products, fish and meat, and nuts may play a crucial role in scavenging ROS, enhancing immune system, suppressing inflammation, and alleviating chronic diseases. Numerous processes in which the phytochemicals are involved suggest the protective role of antioxidants in the pathogenesis of chronic diseases. Taken together, further studies are required to elucidate and gain a better understanding of the degree of ROS production and the types of ROS in relation to diet-induced metabolic ailments.

Competing Interests
The authors declare that there is no conflict of interest regarding the publication of this paper.

B. L. Tan, M. E. Norhaizan, *Nutrients and Oxidative Stress: Biochemistry Aspects and Pharmacological Insights*, SpringerBriefs in Food, Health, and Nutrition, https://doi.org/10.1007/978-3-031-75319-0

Index